T0256071

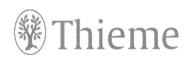

Synopsis of Hand Surgery

Dawn LaPorte, MD
Professor
Department of Orthopaedic Surgery
Johns Hopkins University School of Medicine
Baltimore, Maryland, USA

289 illustrations

Thieme
New York • Stuttgart • Delhi • Rio de Janeiro

Library of Congress Cataloging-in-Publication Data
is available with the publisher

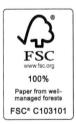

FSC
www.fsc.org
100%
Paper from well-managed forests
FSC® C103101

© 2021. Thieme. All rights reserved.

Thieme Medical Publishers, Inc.
333 Seventh Avenue, New York, NY 10001 USA
+1 800 782 3488, customerservice@thieme.com

Cover design: Thieme Publishing Group
Typesetting by DiTech Process Solutions, India

Printed in USA by King Printing Company, Inc. 5 4 3 2 1

ISBN 978-1-68420-076-4

Also available as an e-book:
eISBN 978-1-68420-077-1

I would like to dedicate this book to my children, Sydney, Zachary, and Cooper, and my husband Paul for their infinite support, love, and patience. I would also like to dedicate the book to my parents, Jere and Michael Mitzner, for their unwavering encouragement and for instilling the love of learning and teaching in their children. Finally, I would like to dedicate this book to all of the Johns Hopkins Orthopedic Surgery residents for their inspiration and spirit of inquiry. Without these individuals, I would not be where I am today!

Dawn LaPorte, MD

Contents

Contents

Videos

Video 2.1 Hand examination.

Video 8.1 Distal radius approach.
   Contributed by Helen Hui-Chou, MD.

Video 18.1 Endoscopic carpal tunnel approach.
   Contributed by Helen Hui-Chou, MD.

Preface

The specialty of hand surgery in the United States originated in the early 20th century during World Wars I and II. Sterling Bunnell served as a surgeon in World War I and recognized that hand injuries were not receiving adequate care. Norman Kirk, Chief of Surgery at Walter Reed National Military Medical Center, was appointed as Army Surgeon General by President Franklin D. Roosevelt during World War II. Kirk and Bunnell were friends and Kirk advocated for Bunnell to be appointed as special civilian consultant to the Secretary of War. Kirk and Bunnell organized nine military hospitals to specialize in the treatment of hand injuries, combining the expertise from orthopaedic, plastic, general, vascular, and neurosurgery to provide a multidisciplinary approach to care of the upper extremity.

This text, *Synopsis of Hand Surgery*, provides an overview of hand surgery, encompassing the important multidisciplinary approach to optimal care of bone and soft tissue conditions in the hand and wrist as emphasized by Bunnell.

Common and more challenging hand and wrist conditions are included with comprehensive information presented in highly illustrated chapters with an easy-to-read bullet point format. The important foundation topics of anatomy, clinical examination, and radiology of the hand and wrist are presented at the start of the book and emphasized throughout. We have also provided some supplementary videos to help the reader understand the details of clinical examination and add to the overall comprehension of the written dialogue.

Synopsis of Hand Surgery should serve as a comprehensive resource on hand for medical students, junior residents in orthopaedic and plastic surgery, and emergency medicine, family practice, and medicine and pediatric physicians.

All of the chapters have been authored by academic hand and upper extremity surgeons or radiologists (Chapter 4 Advanced Imaging). This book was envisioned to be a "go-to" resource for physicians diagnosing and treating conditions of the hand and wrist. It is a pleasure to see *Synopsis of Hand Surgery* completed. We hope it serves its intended purpose and that you enjoy reading the book and that it provides solutions as you care for and help patients with hand symptoms.

Dawn LaPorte, MD

Contributors

Joshua M. Abzug, MD
Associate Professor
Departments of Orthopedics and Pediatrics
University of Maryland School of Medicine;
Director
University of Maryland Brachial Plexus Practice
Director of Pediatric Orthopedics
University of Maryland Medical Center;
Deputy Surgeon-in-Chief
University of Maryland Children's Hospital;
Director and Founder
Camp Open Arms
Timonium, Maryland, USA

Hisham Awan, MD
Orthopaedic Surgeon
The Ohio State University
Wexner Medical Center
Columbus, Ohio, USA

David J. Bozentka, MD
Associate Professor of Orthopaedic Surgery
Chief of the Hand Surgery Section
Department of Orthopaedic Surgery
Hospital of the University of Pennsylvania
Philadelphia, Pennsylvania, USA

Adnan N. Cheema, MD
Resident Physician
Department of Orthopedic Surgery
Hospital of the University of Pennsylvania
Philadelphia, Pennsylvania, USA

Helen Hui-Chou, MD
Assistant Professor
Division of Hand Surgery
Department of Orthopaedic Surgery
University of Miami Miller School of Medicine
Miami, Florida, USA

Anthony F. Colon, MD
Resident
Department of Plastic and Reconstructive Surgery
New Jersey Medical School
Rutgers University
Springfield, New Jersey, USA

Laura M. Fayad, MD
Professor of Radiology, Orthopaedic Surgery, and
    Oncology
Chief of Musculoskeletal Imaging
Director of Translational Research for Advanced
    Imaging
Johns Hopkins University School of
    Medicine
Baltimore, Maryland, USA

Aviram M. Giladi, MD
Research Director
The Curtis National Hand Center
MedStar Union Memorial Hospital
Baltimore, Maryland, USA

Benjamin K. Gundlach, MD
Resident
Department of Orthopaedic Surgery
University of Michigan
Ann Arbor, Michigan, USA

Jessica B. Hawken, MD
Resident
MedStar Union Memorial Hospital
Baltimore, Maryland, USA

Danielle A. Hogarth, BS
Clinical Research Coordinator
Department of Orthopaedics and Pediatrics
University of Maryland School of Medicine
Baltimore, Maryland, USA

Brittany Homcha, MD
Resident
Department of Orthopaedics and
    Rehabilitation
Penn State Milton S. Hershey Medical Center
Hershey, Pennsylvania, USA

John Ingari, MD
Director
Orthopaedic Surgery Residency Program
Sinai Hospital
Baltimore, Maryland, USA

Contributors

Ryan Katz, MD
Plastic and Reconstructive Surgery
The Curtis National Hand Center
MedStar Union Memorial Hospital
Baltimore, Maryland, USA

Michael W. Kessler, MD, MPH
Chief, Department of Orthopedic Surgery
Division of Hand Surgery
MedStar Georgetown University Hospital
Washington, DC, USA

R. Timothy Kreulen, MD
Resident
Department of Orthopaedic Surgery
Johns Hopkins University School of Medicine
Baltimore, Maryland, USA

Hannah C. Langdell, MD
Plastic Surgery Resident
Division of Plastic, Reconstructive, Maxillofacial
    and Oral Surgery
Duke University Medical Center
Durham, North Carolina, USA

Dawn LaPorte, MD
Professor
Department of Orthopaedic Surgery
Johns Hopkins University School of Medicine
Baltimore, Maryland, USA

Jeffrey N. Lawton, MD
Service Chief
Clinical Associate Professor, Orthopedic
    Surgery
Associate Professor, Plastic Surgery
Hand and Upper Extremity
University of Michigan
Ann Arbor, Michigan, USA

Cory Lebowitz, DO
Department of Orthopedic Surgery
Rowan University School of Osteopathic Medicine
Stratford, New Jersey, USA

Laura Lewallen, MD
Hand and Upper Extremity Fellow
Plastic and Reconstructive Surgery
Johns Hopkins University School of Medicine
Baltimore, Maryland, USA

Scott D. Lifchez, MD
Associate Professor of Plastic Surgery and
    Orthopedic Surgery
Johns Hopkins University School of Medicine
Baltimore, Maryland, USA

James S. Lin, MD
Clinical Instructor
Department of Orthopaedics
The Ohio State University
Columbus, Ohio, USA

Viviana Serra López, MD, MS
Resident Physician
Department of Orthopedic Surgery
Hospital of the University of Pennsylvania
Philadelphia, Pennsylvania, USA

Eric Lukosius, MD
Resident
Department of Orthopaedics and Rehabilitation
Penn State Milton S. Hershey Medical Center
Hershey, Pennsylvania, USA

Jonas L. Matzon, MD
Associate Professor
Rothman Orthopaedics
Department of Orthopaedic Surgery
Thomas Jefferson University
Sydney Kimmel Medical College
Philadelphia, Pennsylvania, USA

Roshan T. Melvani, MD
Clinical Fellow
Department of Shoulder and Elbow Surgery
Foundation for Orthopaedic Research and Education
Florida Orthopaedic Institute
Tampa, Florida, USA

Jay L. Mottla, MD
Resident
Department of Orthopaedic Surgery
MedStar Georgetown University Hospital
Washington, DC, USA

Suresh K. Nayar, MD
Resident
Department of Orthopaedics
Johns Hopkins University School of Medicine
Baltimore, Maryland, USA

Manas Nigam, MD
Chief Resident
Department of Plastic and Reconstructive Surgery
MedStar Georgetown University Hospital
Washington, DC, USA

Kevin O'Malley, MD
Resident
Department of Orthopaedic Surgery
MedStar Georgetown University Hospital
Washington, DC, USA

Mitchell A. Pet, MD
Assistant Professor of Plastic Surgery
Department of Plastic and Reconstructive Surgery
Washington University in St. Louis School of
    Medicine
St. Louis, Missouri, USA

Tyler Pidgeon, MD
Assistant Professor
Division of Hand, Upper Extremity, and
    Microvascular Surgery
Department of Orthopaedic Surgery
Duke University Medical Center
Durham, North Carolina, USA

Noah Raizman, MD, MFA
Assistant Clinical Professor
George Washington University
Washington, DC, USA

Samir Sabharwal, MD, MPH
Resident
Department of Orthopaedic Surgery
Johns Hopkins University School of Medicine
Baltimore, Maryland, USA

Richard Samade, MD, PhD
Resident
Department of Orthopaedics
The Ohio State University
Columbus, Ohio, USA

Jonathan Samet, MD
Assistant Professor of Radiology
Section Head of Musculoskeletal Imaging
Department of Medical Imaging
Ann & Robert H. Lurie Children's Hospital of
    Chicago
Northwestern University Feinberg School of
    Medicine
Chicago, Illinois, USA

Julie B. Samora, MD, PhD
Clinical Associate Professor
Department of Orthopaedics
Nationwide Children's Hospital
The Ohio State University
Columbus, Ohio, USA

Eric Schafer, MD
Resident
Department of Orthopedic Surgery
University of Michigan
Ann Arbor, Michigan, USA

Nicole Schroeder, MD
Academy Chair in Orthopaedic Surgery
UCSF Academy of Medical Educators;
Associate Professor
Department of Orthopaedic Surgery
UCSF School of Medicine
San Francisco, California, USA

Michael S. Shear, MD
The Curtis National Hand Center
MedStar Union Memorial Hospital
Baltimore, Maryland, USA

Lauren Lee Smith, MD
Orthopaedic Resident
Department of Orthopaedics
University of Minnesota
Minneapolis, Minnesota, USA

Contributors

Sophia Anne Strike, MD
Assistant Professor
Department of Orthopedic Surgery
Johns Hopkins University School of Medicine
Baltimore, Maryland, USA

Erica Taylor, MD
Orthopaedic Surgeon
Department of Orthopaedics
Duke University School of Medicine
Wake Forest, North Carolina, USA

Kenneth F. Taylor, MD
Professor
Department of Orthopaedics and Rehabilitation
Penn State Milton S. Hershey Medical Center
Hershey, Pennsylvania, USA

Alexandra Tilt, MD
Resident
Division of Plastic and Reconstructive Surgery
Georgetown Universe School of Medicine
Washington, DC, USA

Molly Vora, MA
Medical Student
Boston University School of Medicine
Boston, Massachusetts, USA

Ariel Williams, MD
Assistant Professor
Department of Orthopedic Surgery
University of Minnesota Medical School
Minneapolis, Minnesota, USA

Carson F. Woodbury, MPhil
Medical Student
Johns Hopkins University School of Medicine
Baltimore, Maryland, USA

1 Anatomy and Approaches

Jessica B. Hawken and Aviram M. Giladi

Abstract
Anatomic considerations are a critical aspect of preoperative planning for all surgical procedures; however, nowhere is it more important than in the hand, wrist, and forearm. The relatively superficial location of critical structures including tendons, nerves, and vessels cannot be underestimated or overlooked. This chapter will review anatomy, incisional considerations, and specific approaches for the hand, wrist, and forearm.

Keywords: Anatomy, approaches, surgical planning, surgical exposures

I. Hand

A. Anatomic Compartments

- Thenar: Median, recurrent motor branch nerve
  - Abductor pollicis brevis
  - Flexor pollicis brevis (deep fibers innervated by deep branch of ulnar nerve)
  - Opponens pollicis
- Adductor: Ulnar nerve
  - Adductor pollicis
- Hypothenar: Ulnar nerve
  - Abductor digiti minimi
  - Flexor digiti minimi
  - Opponens digiti minimi
- Interosseous: Ulnar nerve
  - Dorsal interossei (four)
  - Volar interossei (three)
- Lumbricals: 1st and 2nd median nerves, 3rd and 4th deep branch of ulnar nerve
  - 1st and 2nd are unipennate
  - 3rd and 4th are bipennate
  - These muscles originate on the flexor digitorum profundus (FDP) tendons

B. Nerves

- Median
  - Recurrent motor branch
  - Palmar cutaneous branch (branches off the main trunk of the nerve proximal to the carpal tunnel but innervates the palm)
- Ulnar
  - Ulnar motor and ulnar sensory split within Guyon's canal

C. Vasculature

- Superficial palmar arch—continuation of ulnar artery
  - Common digital arteries to index, middle, ring, and small fingers arise from superficial arch
  - Split into proper palmar digital arteries, supplying ulnar side of index finger as well as ulnar and radial arteries to middle, ring, and small fingers
- Deep palmar arch—continuation of radial artery
  - Princeps pollicis branch supplying thumb
  - Radial-side digital artery of index finger

D. Incisional Considerations

- Volar: Avoid deep creases on digits, cross creases at approximately 90-degree angle (Bruner) with the incision running diagonally across the skin in between creases to avoid contracture.
  - Incisions less than 90 degrees may cause skin necrosis of the corner.
  - Avoid travelling too dorsal/lateral while creating the angle to avoid crossing the neurovascular bundles that could be damaged when elevating the flap.
- Dorsal: Often can use smaller incisions due to mobile nature of skin, can be vertical, horizontal, or curved with appropriate skin bridges.
- Fingers can be approached dorsally, volarly, or midaxially.
  - If midaxial, it is best to place the incision at the junction of the glabrous and non-glabrous skin.

E. Approaches

1. Nail Bed

- The nail bed is exposed by bluntly removing the nail plate from the underlying sterile matrix with a noncutting instrument such as a freer.
- Longitudinal incisions in the eponychial fold can be made at the proximal corners radially or ulnarly to expose the proximal nail bed and germinal matrix (▶ Fig. 1.1).

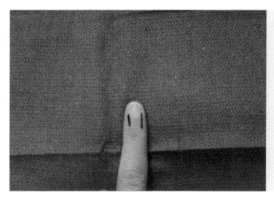

Fig. 1.1 Approach to nail bed.

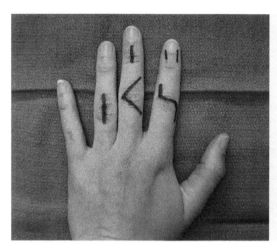

Fig. 1.2 Examples of several dorsal approaches to the proximal and distal interphalangeal joints.

2. Interphalangeal Joints

- Dorsal: A variety of incisions can be used, including straight, curved, S-type, H-type, and chevron (▶ Fig. 1.2).
  - At the distal interphalangeal joint, the germinal matrix is 1 mm distal to the insertion of the extensor tendon, and both are relatively superficial under the skin.
  - The extensor mechanism dictates the approach at the proximal interphalangeal joint. Care should be taken to protect the central slip as it inserts onto the middle phalanx, and the lateral bands.
    - Dorsal approach between the central slip and the lateral bands.
    - Lateral exposure to the joint achieved by freeing the lateral bands and retracting them dorsally.
    - Extensile approach by incising the lateral bands with subsequent repair.
    - The entire extensor mechanism can be removed via the Chamay approach of a distally based V-shaped flap.
- Volar: Zig-zag (aka Bruner) incision through skin to expose the flexor tendon sheath (▶ Fig. 1.3).
  - The pulley overlying the joint is incised longitudinally.
    - Do not incise A2 or A4 pulley whenever possible.
  - The flexor tendons are retracted radially or ulnarly.
  - For more exposure, the split in the superficialis tendon may be carried proximally to allow for more retraction of the profundus tendon.
  - The collateral ligament attachments to the volar plate are incised and the volar plate is mobilized to expose bone.
  - Joint hyperextension exposes articular surfaces.
- Midlateral: Longitudinal incision along midlateral aspect of finger (use the most dorsal aspect of the proximal or distal phalangeal creases as landmarks).
  - The fat overlying the interphalangeal joints is thin; use superficial dissection to avoid incising the joint itself unintentionally.
  - Dissection is carried down the midline of the finger with a slight volar angle.
    - Neurovascular bundle is contained in the volar flap.
  - The flaps can be elevated to expose volarly or dorsally.

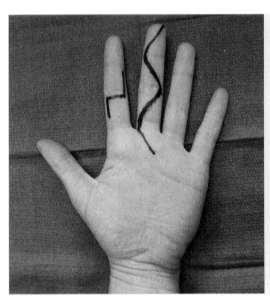

Fig. 1.3 Examples of volar Bruner incision.

3. Metacarpophalangeal Joints

- Gently curved or straight incision centered over the joint. Radially curve over index finger metacarpophalangeal joint (MCPJ) and ulnarly curve over the small finger MCPJ.
  - Avoid undermining skin when creating curved flaps.

4. Metacarpals

- Palpation identifies the metacarpal shaft and overlying extensor tendons (▶ Fig. 1.4).
- The initial incision should be superficial and avoid the tendon.
  - Juncturae tendinae may cross the field and should be protected.
  - If approaching two metacarpals, the incision should be placed between the two.
- To approach the metacarpal, the periosteum of the metacarpal is split and lifted radially and ulnarly, elevating the attached interossei muscles with the flap.

II. Wrist/Forearm

A. Anatomic Compartments

- Carpal tunnel
  - Flexor digitorum profundus tendons
  - Flexor digitorum superficialis tendons
  - Flexor pollicus longus tendon
  - Median nerve
- Guyon's canal
  - Ulnar artery
  - Ulnar nerve

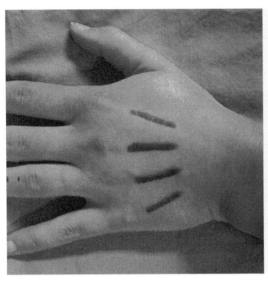

Fig. 1.4 Dorsal approach to the metacarpals.

- Superficial volar forearm: Median nerve
  - Pronator teres
  - Flexor carpi radialis (FCR)
  - Palmaris longus
  - Flexor carpi ulnaris
  - Flexor digitorum superficialis
- Deep volar: Median nerve
  - Flexor digitorum profundus (one half of the innervation from ulnar nerve)
  - Flexor pollicis longus
  - Pronator quadratus
- Dorsal forearm: Radial nerve
  - Abductor pollicis longus
  - Extensor pollicis brevis
  - Extensor pollicis longus
  - Extensor digitorum communis
  - Extensor indicis proprius
  - Extensor digiti quinti
  - Extensory carpi ulnaris
  - Supinator
- Mobile wad: Radial nerve
  - Brachioradialis
  - Extensor carpi radialis longus
  - Extensor carpi radialis brevis

B. Incisional Considerations

- Wrist flexor crease should be treated as palmar creases; do not cross longitudinally.

C. Approaches

1. Carpal Tunnel

- Fibro-osseous tunnel containing the median nerve and nine flexor tendons.
- Borders: Transverse carpal ligament (roof), carpus (floor), hook of hamate and pisiform (ulnar), and scaphoid/trapezium (radial).
- The cardinal line of Kaplan is used to determine the distal border of the tunnel.
  - Base of the first web space parallel to proximal palmar crease toward hook of hamate (▶ Fig. 1.5).
- The location of the distal tip of the fourth metacarpal when flexed to the palm is the longitudinal axis of the incision.
  - Ulnar based incision protects median nerve.
- Incision is carried from the intersection of the longitudinal and perpendicular Cardinal line of Kaplan proximal to the wrist in limited or extensile fashion.
- Dissect through the subcutaneous fat to expose longitudinally oriented superficial palmar fascia.
- Split the fibers of the superficial palmar fascia to expose the deeper transverse fibers of the transverse carpal ligament that are then released:
  - The median nerve is directly underneath this fascia and care should be taken during its release.
  - The distal extent of the incision is reached when yellow-colored palmar fat is seen; beyond this the palmar arch is at risk.
  - The proximal extent is palpable and generally at the level of the distal wrist crease
- The recurrent motor branch of the median nerve is at risk with this approach.
  - Its location and course are variable from person to person and can be pre-, intra-, or post-transverse carpal ligament.

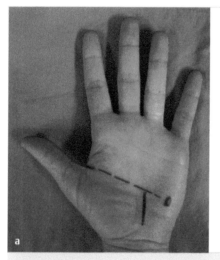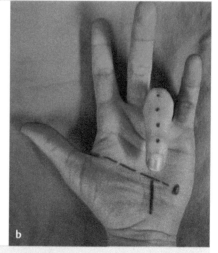

Fig. 1.5 Demonstration of (a) the cardinal line of Kaplan and (b) the axis of the ring finger demonstrating the approach to the carpal tunnel.

D. Guyon's Canal

- Fibro-osseous tunnel that contains the ulnar neurovascular bundle.
- Borders: Volar carpal ligament (roof), transverse carpal ligament (floor), pisiform (ulnar), and hook of hamate (radial).
- The diagonal incision is halfway between the palpable pisiform and hook of hamate with extension along the radial border of the flexor carpi ulnaris tendon as it inserts on the pisiform (▶ Fig. 1.6).
- Incise the fascia along the radial border of the tendon to mobilize it ulnarly.
- The nerve and artery are deep and radial to this tendon; trace them distally until they dive deep to the volar carpal ligament.
- Incise the volar carpal ligament radial to the pisiform.
- The ligament must be released to the extent of the fibrous arch of the hypothenar musculature originating from the hook of the hamate to ensure adequate decompression of the nerve.

1. Volar Approach to Radius (FCR Approach)

- Identify the palpable FCR and begin the incision directly over the tendon (▶ Fig. 1.7).
- The tendon sheath is opened in line with the incision on the radial border.
  - The palmar cutaneous branch of the median nerve runs along the ulnar border of the FCR tendon, and originates from the main median nerve trunk approximately 5 cm proximal to the wrist joint.
- The tendon is retracted ulnarly and the floor of the sheath is opened sharply to expose the area between the flexor tendons and the pronator quadratus.
- Separate flexor pollicus longus from pronator quadratus, and sharply dissect pronator quadratus from the bone in a subperiosteal fashion.

2. Dorsal Approach to Radius

- An 8 cm longitudinal incision starts 3 cm proximal to the wrist joint at the midway point between the palpable radial and ulnar styloids.

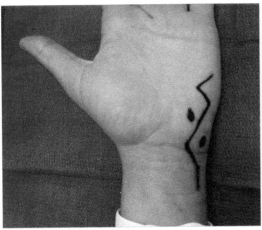

Fig. 1.6 Bruner incision for Guyon's canal. The superior circle is the hook of the hamate, the inferior the palpable pisiform.

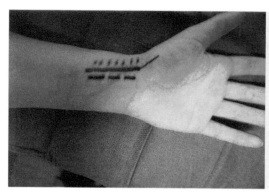

Fig. 1.7 The flexor carpi radialis (FCR) approach to the radius; dotted line is the radial artery, solid is the palpable FCR tendon, and dashed is the palpable palmaris longus tendon.

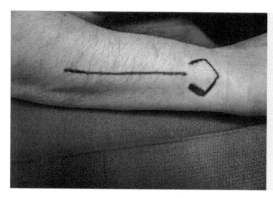

Fig. 1.8 Palpate the ulnar head and shaft to identify the landmarks for the subcutaneous approach to the ulna.

- Under the subcutaneous dissection lies the extensor retinaculum containing the six dorsal compartments of the wrist.
- The fourth compartment is entered sharply through the extensor retinaculum, which should be preserved for repair.
  - This contains the extensor digitorum communis and the extensor indicis proprius.
- The dorsal radiocarpal ligament and the joint capsule are then exposed via ulnar retraction of the tendons, and then the joint can be incised.

3. Subcutaneous Approach to Ulna

- Identify the ulnar head and styloid distally, and the ulnar shaft and tip of the olecranon proximally (▶ Fig. 1.8).
- Begin the incision at the level of the ulnar head distal to the ulnar styloid along the ulnar shaft with the forearm in neutral rotation.
- The ulnar shaft is subcutaneous; the length of the incision is determined by the amount of exposure needed.

Suggested Readings

Bain GI, Pourgiezis N, Roth JH. Surgical approaches to the distal radioulnar joint. Tech Hand Up Extrem Surg. 2007; 11(1):51–56–Review. PubMed PMID: 17536525

Diaz-Garcia R, Waljee JF. Current management of metacarpal fractures. Hand Clin. 2013; 29(4):507–518

Henry AK. Extensile Exposure. 2nd ed. Edinburgh: E&S Livingstone; 1966

Kaplan EB. Functional and Surgical Anatomy of the Hand. 2nd ed. Philadelphia: JB Lippincott; 1965

König PS, Hage JJ, Bloem JJ, Prosé LP. Variations of the ulnar nerve and ulnar artery in Guyon's canal: a cadaveric study. J Hand Surg Am. 1994; 19(4):617–622

McClelland WB, Jr, McClinton MA. Proximal interphalangeal joint injection through a volar approach: anatomic feasibility and cadaveric assessment of success. J Hand Surg Am. 2013; 38(4):733–739

2 History and Examination of the Hand

Carson F. Woodbury and Laura Lewallen

Abstract
Careful physical examination combined with a targeted history is the essential first step in the practice of hand surgery. This chapter describes key elements of history in the hand surgery patient and then proceeds through each component of the hand examination: inspection, vascular assessment, sensation, palpation, range of motion, ligament stability, and musculotendinous function. The core maneuvers of the hand examination are defined and illustrated with photographs and videos. A sample documentation is also provided for a normal hand examination.

Keywords: Hand examination, upper extremity examination, physical examination, evaluation of injury, disease history

I. History

- History of the present illness
  - First line should include hand dominance and occupation:
    - Sheds light on acute injuries and stress injuries.
    - Helps determine time available for recovery from disease/injury or surgery if needed and guides the priority of reconstructive procedures.
  - Injury history
    - Mechanism: What (the instrument) and how (slice, crush, tear, etc.).
    - Posture of hand at time of injury.
    - Where: Can help determine degree of contamination (factory, toolshed, farm, combat).
    - When: Helps determine potential ischemia time, likelihood of infection, and options for treatment.
    - Prior treatment: Tetanus, wound cleansing, antibiotics, tourniquet, and treatment of amputated part(s).
  - Symptoms
    - "Where does it hurt?"
    - Cold part, loss of sensation, paresthesias, weakness, loss of coordination, dislocation, clicking, snapping, and popping.
    - Classify by: Location, onset, course, severity/quality, alleviating factors, exacerbating factors, associated symptoms, and prior experience.
    - Effect on daily life, occupation, and hobbies.
    - Confirm that described symptoms are limited to single body part or associated with active systemic disease.
  - Pregnancy or last menstrual period for reproductive-age female.
  - "When did you last eat or drink something?" (trauma patient).
  - Last tetanus immunization.
- Past medical history, with special attention to the following:
  - Major medical conditions affecting wound healing, (e.g., diabetes mellitus).
  - Major cardiac, pulmonary, or renal disease.

- ○ Rheumatologic disease.
- ○ Immunocompromised: HIV, transplant, leukemia, etc.
- Past surgical history, with special attention to the following:
  - ○ Prior operations in region of injury/disease.
  - ○ Complications with anesthesia or bleeding.
- Medications, with special attention to the following:
  - ○ Steroids.
  - ○ Immunosuppressants.
  - ○ Anticoagulants.
- Allergies, with special attention to the following:
  - ○ Antibiotics.
  - ○ Latex.
  - ○ Shellfish may raise concern for iodine allergy.
- Family history, with special attention to the following:
  - ○ Heart disease.
  - ○ Rheumatologic disease.
  - ○ Dupuytren's disease.
  - ○ Congenital conditions.
  - ○ Complications with anesthesia or bleeding.
- Social history:
  - ○ Occupation.
  - ○ Hobbies/sports.
  - ○ Substance use.
  - ○ Intravenous drug use.

II. Principles of Complete Examination

- Basic principles apply:
  - ○ Be systematic and thorough.
  - ○ Remove dressings, clothing, and jewelry including from the contralateral side to ensure complete exposure.
  - ○ Adequate lighting is essential, especially if infection is suspected and erythema must be delineated.
  - ○ Plain film radiographs in three views (anteroposterior, lateral, and oblique) are useful in most clinical visits and essential in emergency department evaluations.
  - ○ If anesthesia is required for a complete examination, assess sensation first and motor if possible.
  - ○ All findings should be compared to the contralateral side.
- An experienced examiner may pick and choose the necessary maneuvers, but care should be taken by trainees when skipping portions of the examination to ensure no injury or evidence of disease is missed.
- At minimum, a complete examination should include the following:
  - ○ Inspection
  - ○ Vascular assessment
  - ○ Sensation
  - ○ Palpation
  - ○ Range of motion
  - ○ Musculotendinous/neuromotor function

III. Inspection

- Injury
  - Is skin closed and intact?
  - Degree of contamination
  - Foreign bodies
  - Are deep structures visible?
- Deformities
  - Angulation
  - Malrotation of fingers: Tips should point to scaphoid tubercle when flexed at meta-carpophalangeal (MP) and proximal interphalangeal (PIP) joints
  - Visible masses
  - Drawings or photographs are useful for communication and surgical planning (obtain patient permission before taking photographs)
- Posture
  - Resting cascade of fingers (▶ Fig. 2.1)
    - Flexion of fingers: Small > ring > middle > index
  - Motion at rest, e.g., tremors
- Swelling
  - Localized, diffuse within a region, or generalized across body?
    - Fusiform swelling suggests flexor tenosynovitis
    - Look for loss of finger creases
  - Restricted by anatomy?
    - Palmar inflammation may present as dorsal swelling due to the tightness of the palmar fascia
    - Apparent delineation along borders of forearm compartments suggesting a possible compartment syndrome
- Skin
  - Scars from prior injury or surgery
  - Skin color and distribution of color
    - Erythema suggests infection, inflammation/arthritis flare, or gout.
    - Delineate borders of erythema with pen or skin marker and note the time.

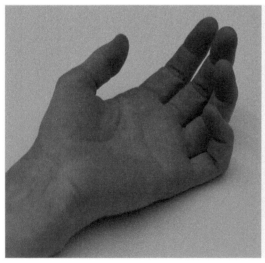

Fig. 2.1 Resting cascade of fingers. Flexion is greatest in the small finger and decreases in each more radial finger.

- – Streaking may be seen with infection.
- – Pale color suggests arterial insufficiency.
- – Purple/dark red color suggests venous insufficiency or contusion.
  - ○ Lesions
    - – Small can be meaningful; (e.g., paint gun injury may produce tiny puncture wound but causes tremendous inflammation and destruction in the hand).
    - – Ulcers.
    - – Soft tissue infarcts.
    - – Neoplasms.
    - – Calcinosis.
  - ○ Perspiration: If present, are there areas that are dry?
- • Nails
  - ○ Clubbing: Associated with systemic disease but may also be benign.
  - ○ Paronychia: Infection of the nailfold.
  - ○ Koilonychia: Spoon-shaped nails, associated with iron deficiency.
- • Wasting
  - ○ Unilateral vs. bilateral: Suggests local or systemic pathology, respectively.
  - ○ Which muscles?
    - – Thenar suggests median nerve pathology.
    - – Interosseous or hypothenar suggests ulnar nerve pathology.
  - ○ Measure girth
- • Observing pediatric patients
  - ○ Young children who have difficulty cooperating with the examination may be encouraged to play with age-appropriate toys and watched closely.
  - ○ Alternatively, bouncing a ball back and forth between examiner and child provides abundant information on range of motion, dexterity, and reaction time.
    - – First, ask child to catch with right hand. Bounce to different heights and distances from body. Next, ask child to switch to left hand.
  - ○ Data gleaned from careful observation can target the necessary provocative tests to confirm or rule out diagnoses.

IV. Vascular Assessment

- • Vascular system is assessed first in an emergency department evaluation to quickly determine if there is ischemia and a more urgent evaluation and treatment are warranted.
- • Brief assessment
  - ○ Skin color (see above): Are digits pink and warm or pale or blue or dusky?
  - ○ Palpate skin temperature, comparing to other digits and contralateral hand.
  - ○ Palpate radial and ulnar artery pulses (if not palpable, check Doppler).
  - ○ Capillary refill should be <2 seconds beneath the fingernails.
- • If ischemia is suspected
  - ○ Pencil Doppler can be placed on the pad of each fingertip to listen for distal pulses.
  - ○ Pulse oximeter can be applied to a digit.
  - ○ Fingertip can be pricked with 25-gauge needle. Normal finger will show bright red capillary bleeding.
- • Allen test (▶ Fig. 2.2, **Video 2.1**):
  - ○ Assesses for patency of palmar arterial arch.

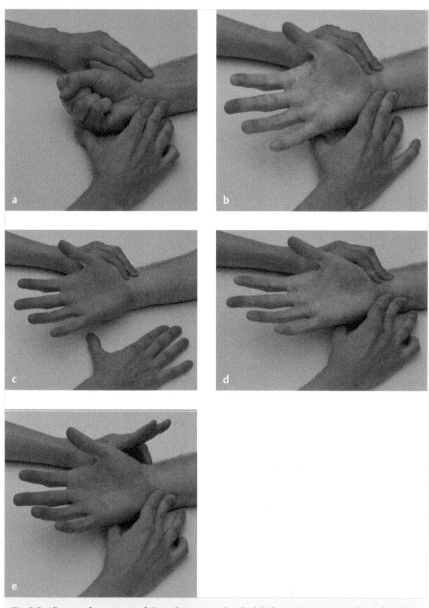

Fig. 2.2 Allen test for patency of the palmar arterial arch. **(a)** The patient squeezes his or her hand into a fist, and the examiner firmly compresses the radial and ulnar arteries at the wrist. **(b)** Patient opens hand to reveal exsanguinated palm. **(c)** Release pressure on the ulnar artery and watch for full perfusion of the hand. **(d, e)** Repeat with release of pressure on the radial artery.

- At least one palmar arch is intact in 97% of patients, enabling the entire hand to be perfused by either the radial or the ulnar artery.[1]
    1. Deep arch is usually radial.
    2. Superficial arch is usually ulnar.
- Firmly compress radial and ulnar arteries at wrist. Patient makes repeated tight fists to exsanguinate hand and then relaxes fingers. Release pressure on radial artery and watch for blood to return (refill time). Repeat with release of ulnar artery.
- Normal = <3 seconds with whole hand being perfused.
- Digital Allen's test
    - Assesses for collateral flow between ulnar and radial digital arteries.
    - Compress ulnar and radial side of patient's fingertip and move proximally to exsanguinate finger. Release the radial side and look for return of blood to entire finger (refill time). Repeat with ulnar side.
    - Normal = <3 seconds.

V. Sensation

A. First Principles

- Sensory examination should be completed before anesthesia (if needed to complete examination).
- Based on knowledge of cutaneous innervation by peripheral nerve distributions and dermatomes.
- At minimum, light touch and sharp sense should be documented at the radial and ulnar tip of each digit.
    - Light touch: Cotton swab or examiner's finger.
    - Sharp sense: Broken tip of a wooden cotton swab.
        - Warn patient it should feel sharp but will not hurt.
        - Apply enough pressure to depress the skin slightly but not enough to puncture or draw blood. Be cognizant of elderly patients with thin, fragile skin.
        - Stabilize hand holding the cotton swab against the patient's hand to avoid inadvertently pressing too hard.
- Ideally, light and sharp sense should be assessed in proximal and distal areas supplied by each major nerve and compared to the contralateral side.
- Carefully delineate and document any areas of numbness or diminished sensation.
- Evaluate the effect of hand and extremity position on symptoms.

B. Advanced Sensory Testing

- Two-point discrimination: Static or moving/dynamic
    - Normal static = 6 mm; based on Merkel cells.
    - Normal dynamic = 3 mm; based on Meissner corpuscles.
- Semmes-Weinstein monofilaments: Pressure perception thresholds
    - Record the number of the thinnest filament for which the patient can sense the pressure required to bend the filament.
    - Patient should *not* feel the touch of the unbent filament on the skin.

- Vibration: 30 Hz and 250 Hz tuning forks
  - Recorded as a threshold.
- Temperature: Test tubes containing ice water and water at 40 to 45 °C.
  - Rarely clinically useful, but may be helpful in documenting return of protective sensation following nerve injury.

C. Cervical Examination

- Important to evaluate for cervical root compression or spinal pathology as causes of upper extremity neurologic symptoms.
- Presence of cervical pathology does not exclude peripheral nerve compression or injury; e.g., it is possible to have root compression and carpal tunnel syndrome simultaneously ("double crush").
- Axial load test
  - Assesses nerve root compression.
  - With head in neutral position, press down on the top of the head with moderate pressure.
  - Positive = reproduction of radicular symptoms in the upper extremities.
- Spurling's test (▶ Fig. 2.3, **Video 2.1**)
  - Also known as foraminal compression test, it assesses for stenosis of the vertebral foramina through which cervical nerves pass.
  - Gently rotate neck approximately 20 degrees to affected side and laterally bend neck toward affected side by about 20 degrees. Then apply gentle axial compression.
  - Positive = reproduction of radicular symptoms in the upper extremities.

D. Provocative Tests

- Tinel's sign: Paresthesia or pain in the distribution of the nerve being tested when the area overlying the nerve is tapped firmly.
  - It may be applied to median nerve compression in the carpal tunnel or ulnar nerve compression in the cubital tunnel or Guyon's canal.

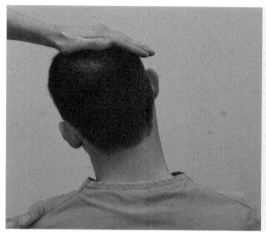

Fig. 2.3 Spurling's test for foraminal compression. Gently rotate the neck 20 degrees to affected side and laterally bend neck toward affected side. Then apply gentle axial compression. Reproduction of radicular symptoms in the upper extremity is a positive test and indicates stenosis of the vertebral foramen/foramina.

- After nerve injury, the most distant point of paresthesia represents the furthest extent of nerve regeneration; Tinel's sign can be followed as a marker of nerve recovery/regeneration.
- Median nerve pathology
  - Direct compression test (Durkan's test, ▶ Fig. 2.4).
    - Direct compression over the carpal tunnel by the examiner's thumb for 30 seconds.
    - Positive = pain or paresthesia in the median nerve distribution.
  - Phalen's test (▶ Fig. 2.5)
    - Hold wrists in maximum palmar flexion for up to 2 minutes.
    - Positive = pain or paresthesia in the median nerve distribution.

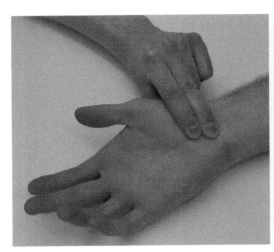

Fig. 2.4 Direct compression test for median nerve compression at the carpal tunnel. A positive test produces pain or paresthesia in the median nerve distribution.

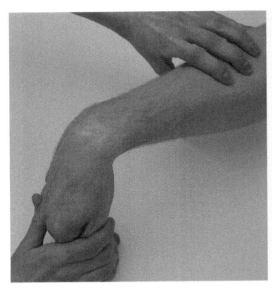

Fig. 2.5 Phalen's test for median nerve compression at the carpal tunnel. The examiner holds the wrist in maximum palmar flexion for up to 2 minutes. A positive test produces pain or paresthesia in the median nerve distribution.

- Ulnar nerve pathology
  - Elbow flexion test
    - Assesses for cubital tunnel syndrome.
    - Supinate forearms and hold elbows in maximum flexion for 60 seconds.
    - Positive = pain or paresthesia in the ulnar nerve distribution.
  - Duchenne's sign
    - Also known as ulnar clawing or intrinsic-minus.
    - Ring and small fingers have hyperextended MP and flexed PIP and distal inter-phalangeal (DIP).
    - Indicates loss of intrinsic function with preservation of flexor digitorum profundus (FDP) from a distal ulnar nerve injury.
  - Froment's test
    - Assesses thumb adduction (ADP).
    - Patient holds a piece of paper or folder between tip of thumb and radial base of the index finger in a lateral/key pinch. Examiner gradually pulls the paper away, encouraging the patient to keep hold of it.
    - Positive = flexion of thumb interphalangeal (IP) joint.
    - Usually combined with Jeanne's sign.
    - May also see hyperextension of index finger DIP and flexion of index finger PIP.
  - Jeanne's sign
    - ADP.
    - Present = patient hyperextends MP joint during lateral/key pinch to "lock" the joint, compensating weak or paralyzed ADP.
  - Wartenberg's sign
    - Assesses palmar interosseous muscles.
    - With hands flat on table, patient is asked to adduct all fingers.
    - Present = inability to adduct small finger.
    - Indicates weak/paralyzed third palmar interosseous resulting in unopposed extensor digiti minimi (EDM).
  - Pitres-Testut sign
    - Assesses second and third dorsal interosseous muscles.
    - With palm flat on table, hyperextend middle finger and deviate it radially and ulnarly.
    - Present = inability to make this motion.

VI. Palpation

- Tenderness/pain
  - "Where does it hurt?" Assess painful areas last.
  - If concern for infection, palpate cervical and axillary lymph nodes.
- Swelling
  - Does it feel edematous?
  - Calcified?
  - Synovial enlargement?
  - Gouty deposits?
  - Effusion?
  - Fluctuance (fluid collection)?
- Masses
  - Well-circumscribed or irregular borders.
  - Mobile or fixed.

- Firm, soft, rubbery, etc.
- Tender or nontender.
- Joints
  - Move proximal to distal or distal to proximal.
  - Support patient's hand with yours and ask them to relax muscles.
  - Feel for tenderness, swellings, crepitus, clicking, and snapping.
  - Thumb carpometacarpal (CMC) grind test (**Video 2.1**)
    - Assesses for CMC arthritis of the thumb.
    - Grasp the patient's thumb with one hand and stabilize the palm with the other. Compress the CMC joint along the axis of the ray and rotate the digit in a cylindrical motion around this axis.
    - Positive = reproduction of pain in the CMC joint of the thumb.

VII. Range of Motion

- Range of motion (ROM)
  - Measured in the posture that permits maximum motion at the joint.
  - Isolate the joint from movement in planes other than the plane being tested.
  - Goniometer (▶ Fig. 2.6): Hinged protractor used to measure joint angle more precisely.
  - Active ROM (patient-initiated movement of a body part) represents the sum of:
    - Musculotendinous function.
    - Joint function with or without pathology.
    - Ligament stability/mobility.
    - Superficial soft tissue pliability.
  - Passive ROM (examiner moves patient's body part) removes musculotendinous function from the equation.
    - Passive ROM frequently greater than active ROM in normal joints.
  - Loss of ROM can be caused by pathology with any of the components of motion.
    - For example, the burned hand may develop skin contractures that limit ROM even if the motor nerves, muscles, and tendons were spared.
  - ROM is described as joint + plane of motion + degrees of motion (▶ Table 2.1).
  - Pain with active and/or passive ROM should be assessed and documented.
    - For example, flexor tendon injury typically produces pain with active motion and passive extension; there is typically no pain during passive joint flexion.

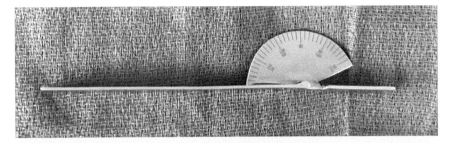

Fig. 2.6 Goniometers are used to measure joint angles precisely.

Table 2.1 Range of motion definitions and approximate normal values

Motion	Definition	Normal ROM[a]	Impaired ROM[b]
Elbow			
Flexion–extension	• Full extension = 0 degree • Flexion = angle between forearm and line extending from the distal humerus	Extension = 0 degree Flexion = 150 degrees	10 degrees 130 degrees
Varus–valgus	• Varus = distal part angled toward midline • Valgus = distal part angled away from midline • Measured as deviation from neutral	Varus = 5 to 10 degrees Valgus = 5 to 10 degrees	n.a.
Forearm			
Pronation–supination	• Neutral position = elbow in 90 degrees flexion, arm adducted to side, forearm rotated to position where extended thumb points cranially • ROM measured as arc deviation from neutral position	Pronation = 75 degrees Supination = 85 degrees	70 degrees 60 degrees
Wrist			
Flexion–extension	• Neutral position = midpoint between flexion and extension • Measured as deviation from neutral	Flexion = 80 degrees Extension = 75 degrees	50 degrees 50 degrees
Radial–ulnar deviation	• Measured as deviation from neutral axis through the middle finger in neutral flexion-extension • Ulnar > radial	Radial = 20 degrees Ulnar = 30 degrees	10 degrees 20 degrees
Thumb			
Flexion–extension	• 0 degree set at position where bones of the ray are in line with each other • Negative values indicate hyperextension • Highly variable	MP = 0 to 50 degrees IP = -10 to 75 degrees	10 to 50 degrees 0 to 70 degrees
Abduction–adduction	• Abduction = movement of the thumb metacarpal out of the plane of the palm • Adduction = movement of the thumb metacarpal into the plane of the palm • Palmar plane = 0 degree	0 to 70 degrees	n.a.

Table 2.1 (*Continued*) Range of motion definitions and approximate normal values

Motion	Definition	Normal ROM[a]	Impaired ROM[b]
Opposition	• Movement across the palm toward the small finger • Requires CMC flexion and pronation, MP flexion, and IP flexion • Impairment defined by maximum distance between thumb IP flexor crease and distal palmar crease over middle finger (normal > 7 cm)	Thumb touches small finger MP or > 7 cm between thumb IP flexor crease and distal palmar crease over middle finger	6 cm
Fingers			
Flexion–extension	• 0 degree set at position where bones of the ray are in line with each other • Negative values indicate hyperextension	MP = −10 to 90 degrees PIP = 0 to 110 degrees DIP = −10 to 80 degrees	−10 to 80 degrees 10 to 90 degrees 10 to 60 degrees
Abduction–adduction	• Abduction = movement away from middle finger • Adduction = movement toward middle finger	0 to 20 degrees	n.a.

[a]Range of motion (ROM) values from Netter's Concise Orthopaedic Anatomy.[2]
[b]Maximum ROM defined as "mild impairment" by legal standard: Guides to the Evaluation of Permanent Impairment, 6th ed.[3] Extension lag values converted to equivalent flexion angle for consistency.
Abbreviations: DIP, distal interphalangeal; IP, interphalangeal; MP, metacarpophalangeal; PIP, proximal interphalangeal.

- Brief ROM examination
  - Ask patient to do the following and demonstrate the motions:
    - Raise both hands with palms facing examiner.
    - Abduct fingers fully.
    - Adduct fingers fully.
    - Flex MP joints, keeping PIP and DIP of the index, middle, ring, and small fingers extended (lumbrical-plus position).
    - Extend MP joints; keeping MP joints extended, flex PIP and DIP of the index, middle, ring, and small fingers.
    - Make fists with thumbs adducted over the folded fingers.
    - Lower hands so forearms are parallel to the floor.
    - Flex and extend wrists fully.
    - Deviate wrists ulnarly and radially.
    - Make two thumbs-up and bring elbows to patient's sides; pronate and supinate fully.
    - Relax hands and arms by patient's sides and extend elbows fully; flex elbows fully, touching hands to shoulders if possible.

- Maneuvers to alter ROM
  - Can be used to determine if limited ROM is due to capsular contracture or soft tissue scarring vs. musculotendinous pathology.
  - Passive wrist flexion causes fingers to extend passively (tenodesis effect).
  - Passive wrist extension causes fingers to flex passively (tenodesis effect).
  - Extrinsic tightness test (▶ Fig. 2.7):
    - Assesses for tightness of extrinsic finger extensors (extensor digitorum, extensor indicis proprius, EDM).
    - Positive = PIP flexion increases when MP is extended (compared with MP flexed).
  - Intrinsic tightness test (▶ Fig. 2.8).
    - Assesses tightness of interosseous and lumbrical muscles.
    - Positive = PIP flexion increases when MP is flexed from 0 degree (compared with MP extended).
    - Bunnell's sign = positive intrinsic tightness test.
  - Lumbrical tightness test.
    - Also known as lumbrical-plus test.
    - Principle: Tight lumbrical muscles overcome dysfunctional FDP and force finger into extension when FDP contracts—called paradoxical movement.
    - Positive = Patient attempts to flex digits, and PIP and DIP extend:

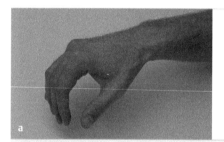
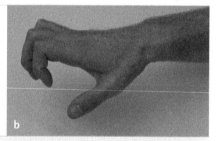

Fig. 2.7 Simulation of the extrinsic tightness test. Proximal interphalangeal (PIP) flexion is less when metacarpophalangeal (MP) joints are flexed **(a)** compared to when MP joints are extended **(b)**.

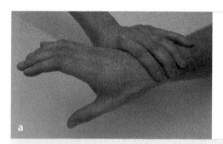
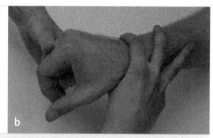

Fig. 2.8 Simulation of the intrinsic tightness test. Proximal interphalangeal (PIP) flexion is less when metacarpophalangeal (MP) joints are extended **(a)** compared to when MP joints are flexed **(b)**.

VIII. Ligament Stability

- Assess stability of a ligament when that ligament is tight:
  - MP collateral ligaments tight in flexion.
  - PIP and DIP ligaments tight in extension.

A. Tests of Radioulnar Ligaments

- Distal radioulnar joint (DRUJ) instability test (**Video 2.1**)
  - Principle: Deep dorsal ligament taut in supination; deep palmar ligament taut in pronation.
  - In full pronation, apply pressure palmarly to distal ulna:
    – Abnormal dorsal movement suggests injury to palmar distal radioulnar ligament.
  - In full supination, apply pressure dorsally to distal ulna:
    – Abnormal palmar movement suggests injury to dorsal distal radioulnar ligament.
- Ulnocarpal abutment test (**Video 2.1**)
  - Assesses for triangular fibrocartilage complex (TFCC) injury and ulnar impaction syndrome (long ulna = ulnar-positive; seen on zero rotation radiographs).
  - With forearm stabilized and thumb on distal ulna, wrist is fully deviated ulnarly; then pronate and supinate the forearm.
  - Positive = ulnar wrist pain, may feel click/pop over ulnocarpal joint.
- Ulnar fovea sign
  - Assesses injury to TFCC, distal radioulnar ligament, and ulnotriquetral ligament.
  - With elbow at approximately 90 degrees flexion, neutral rotation, and neutral wrist, apply pressure with examiner's thumb in a soft spot between ulnar styloid process, pisiform, flexor carpi ulnaris tendon, and the palmar ulnar head (the ulnar fovea).
  - Positive = severe tenderness.
  - Fovea = pit.
- Piano key sign
  - Indicates destructive synovitis of ulnocarpal ligaments,
    – Associated with rheumatoid arthritis,
  - With hand in pronation, examiner places thumb on dorsal ulnar styloid and applies pressure to displace the ulna palmarly. Release of pressure causes the ulna to return to its dorsal subluxed position like a piano key rising after being pressed.

B. Tests of Carpal Ligaments

- Scaphoid shift test (Watson's test) (▶ Fig. 2.9, **Video 2.1**)[4]
  - Assesses for insufficiency of the scapholunate ligament, scaphoid fracture, or scapholunate advanced collapse (SLAC) arthritis.
  - Principle: Radial deviation of wrist produces palmar rotation of the scaphoid.
  - Place thumb over palmar scaphoid tuberosity. Deviate wrist from ulnar to radial while applying pressure to the scaphoid, resisting the palmar rotation.
  - Positive = pain *and* feeling of clunk or give as the scaphoid subluxes over the dorsal rim of the radial head.
- Lunotriquetral ballottement test
  - Assesses lunotriquetral ligament integrity.

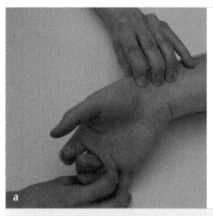
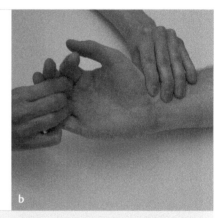

Fig. 2.9 Scaphoid shift test (also known as Watson's test) assesses the scapholunate ligament. **(a)** Place the examiner's thumb over the palmar scaphoid tuberosity. **(b)** Deviate wrist from ulnar to radial while applying pressure to the scaphoid, resisting palmar rotation. Test is positive if the patient experiences pain and the examiner feels a "clunk" or give.

- ○ Keeping patient's forearm pronated, examiner pinches triquetrum and pisiform as a unit between thumb and index with thumb dorsal. The other thumb provides pressure on the dorsal lunate to displace it palmarly.
- ○ Positive = palmar movement and wrist pain.
- ○ Ballottement = palpating anatomy of structures floating in fluid.
- Midcarpal instability test
  - ○ Assesses the joints between the proximal and distal carpal rows.
  - ○ Stabilizing the forearm with examiner's thumb on dorsal midcarpal joint, deviate wrist ulnarly and radially.
  - ○ Positive = pain in midcarpal joint, may have click/pop/clunk.

C. Tests of Finger Ligaments

- Ulnar collateral ligament (UCL) test
  - ○ Assesses UCL of the thumb.
  - ○ With MP fully flexed, deviate thumb radially at the MP joint. Repeat with MP extended.
  - ○ Positive = > 30 degrees radial deviation in both positions or if grossly increased deviation compared with contralateral side.
  - ○ Chronic UCL injury = Gamekeeper's thumb.

IX. Musculotendinous Function

- Loss of musculotendinous function can be caused by injury/disease at any level between the brain and the joint being moved:
  - ○ Cerebral.
  - ○ Spinal.
  - ○ Brachial plexus.
  - ○ Peripheral nerve.

○ Neuromuscular junction.
○ Muscle.
○ Tendon.
○ Tendon insertion.
○ Mechanical obstruction.

A. Motor Examination by Nerve

- Posterior interosseous (radial): Extend index finger and thumb (make a pistol, extensor pollicis longus, extensor pollicis brevis, and extensor indicis proprius).
- Anterior interosseous (median): Touch tips of thumb and index fingers to make a ring (A-okay sign, flexor digitorum profundus to index finger and flexor pollicis longus).
- Recurrent motor branch (median): Oppose thumb to small finger MP joint (opponens pollicis).
- Ulnar: Abduct fingers fully (dorsal interossei, abductor digiti minimi).

B. Strength Testing

- Graded clinically on a scale of 0 to 5 or quantitatively with a dynamometer (▶ Fig. 2.10).
  ○ Dynamometer may be used for grip strength and pinch strength.
- Medical Research Council Scale[5].
  ○ 0 = no contraction of muscle.
  ○ 1 = flicker or trace movement (with active volition).
  ○ 2 = active movement with gravity eliminated (plane parallel to ground).
  ○ 3 = active movement against gravity.
  ○ 4 = active movement against gravity and resistance from examiner.
  ○ 4–/5 = movement against small amount of resistance.
  ○ 4 + /5 = movement against strong resistance.
  ○ 5 = normal power (overcomes examiner's resistance).

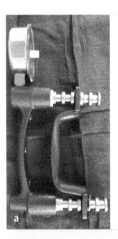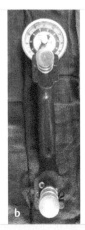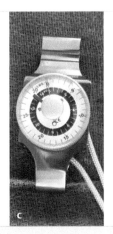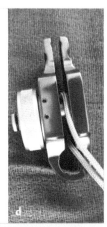

Fig. 2.10 Dynamometers for grip strength (a, b) and pinch strength (c, d).

- Stabilize the joint above the joint being tested.
- Basic assessment of strength:
  - Elbow flexion
  - Elbow extension
  - Wrist flexion
  - Wrist extension
  - MCP extension
  - Opposition pinch strength: Examiner and patient make interlocking rings by pinching their index fingers and thumbs; examiner tries to break patient's ring
  - Finger abduction

C. Testing Individual Musculotendinous Units

- Test a musculotendinous unit in the position where cooperative muscles do not function.
  - For example, extensor digitorum communis (EDC) functions as a wrist extender. To isolate extensor carpi radialis longus (ECRL), extensor carpi radialis brevis (ECRB), and extensor carpi ulnaris (ECU), the patient should make a fist to relax EDC.
- Forearm
  - Pronation: Pronator teres, pronator quadratus
  - Supination: Supinator
- Wrist
  - Wrist flexion: Flexor carpi radialis (FCR), flexor carpi ulnaris (FCU)
    - Keep fingers extended to eliminate minor flexors: FDP, flexor digitorum superficialis (FDS).
  - Wrist extension: ECRL, ECRB, ECU
    - Make fist to eliminate minor extensor: EDC.
  - Wrist ulnar deviation: ECU, FCU
  - Wrist radial deviation: ECRL, ECRB, FCR
- Fingers
  - Finger flexion (isolated)
    - MP: Lumbricals, interossei
    - PIP: FDS. Isolate FDS action in a finger by holding the adjacent fingers in extension. This prevents FDP from being used to flex the test finger. If FDS is intact or partially intact, patient will still be able to flex the PIP of the finger being tested (▶ Fig. 2.11).
    - DIP: FDP. Isolate FDP by blocking PIP flexion in the tested digit (▶ Fig. 2.12).
  - Finger extension
    - MP: EDC. Test by extending MP joints while keeping PIP and DIP flexed.
    - PIP: EDC, lumbricals, interossei.
    - DIP: EDC, lumbricals, interossei.
    - Index finger: Extensor indicis proprius (EIP). Test by making a fist and then straightening index finger completely.
    - Small finger: EDM. Test by making a fist and straightening small finger.
  - Finger abduction: Dorsal interossei (4), 1st and 2nd lumbricals
    - Test the 2nd and 3rd dorsal interossei by placing palm flat on table, hyperextending middle finger to lift it off table, and deviating radially and ulnarly.
    - Pitres-Testut sign = inability to do this, suggestive of ulnar nerve injury.

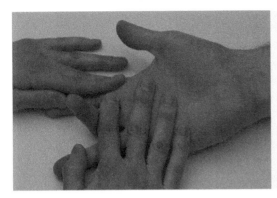

Fig. 2.11 Isolating flexor digitorum superficialis.

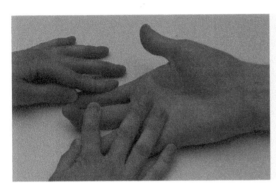

Fig. 2.12 Isolating flexor digitorum profundus.

  - Test the 1st palmar interosseous and the 2nd dorsal interosseous by crossing middle finger over index finger with remaining fingers flat on table.
  ○ Finger adduction: Palmar interossei (3), 3rd and 4th lumbricals.
- Thumb
  ○ Thumb extension: Extensor pollicis longus (EPL), extensor pollicis brevis (EPB).
    - With hand flat on table, lift only thumb off and palpate EPL.
  ○ Thumb flexion: Flexor pollicis longus (FPL), flexor pollicis brevis (FPB).
  ○ Thumb opposition: Abductor pollicis brevis (APB), opponens pollicis (OP).
  ○ Thumb adduction: Adductor pollicis (ADP).
    - Lateral pinch (key pinch) tests thumb adduction.
  ○ Thumb abduction: Abductor pollicis longus (APL), APB.
    - Place dorsum of hand on table and raise thumb to perpendicular. Resist examiner pushing down on thumb (contribution from EPL).

D. Provocative Tests

- Tests for de Quervain's tenosynovitis (inflammation of 1st extensor compartment)
  ○ Finkelstein's test (**Video 2.1**): Examiner flexes the MP joint by pressing on the head of the proximal phalanx:
    - Positive = pain along EPB and APL tendons (1st extensor compartment).

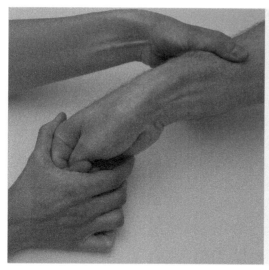

Fig. 2.13 Eichoff's test for de Quervain's tenosynovitis. Patient holds thumb inside the fist and examiner deviates hand ulnarly. Positive test is pain along extensor pollicis brevis (EPB) and abductor pollicis longus (APL) tendons and suggests inflammation of the 1st extensor compartment.

- Eichoff's test (▶ Fig. 2.13, **Video 2.1**): Patient holds thumb inside the fist and examiner deviates hand ulnarly.
    - Positive = pain along EPB and APL tendons.
- Extensor carpi ulnaris synergy test
    - Assesses for ECU tendinitis.
    - In full supination, patient attempts to abduct all fingers while examiner pinches the index and small fingers with enough force to prevent abduction.
    - Positive = pain along ECU tendon (6th dorsal compartment).

X. Documenting a Normal Examination

The following is a sample documentation of a normal examination.
- **Inspection:** Resting cascade of the fingers is present and within normal limits. No obvious deformity, mass, swelling, or skin lesion. No thenar or interosseous atrophy.
- **Vascular:** Skin is pink and warm. 2 + radial and ulnar pulses bilaterally. Capillary refill brisk.
- **Sensation:** Light touch and sharp sense grossly intact in a median, radial, and ulnar nerve distribution bilaterally. No numbness or paresthesia.
- **Joints:** No tenderness to palpation, crepitus, or effusions in the wrist, CMC, MP, or IP joints. No apparent ligamentous laxity.
- **Range of motion:** See ▶ Table 2.2.
- **Motor:** Musculocutaneous nerve, radial nerve, posterior interosseous nerve (PIN), anterior interosseous nerve (AIN), recurrent motor branch of median nerve, and ulnar nerve functionally intact (▶ Table 2.3).

Table 2.2 Range of motion documentation

Left (degrees)	Motion	Right (degrees)
60	Wrist flexion	50
60	Wrist extension	60
0–90	Thumb flexion–extension MP	0–80
–30–80	Thumb flexion–extension IP	–30–80
Full	Thumb abduction–adduction	Full
Full	Thumb opposition	Full
–10–90	Finger flexion–extension MP	–10–90
0–100	Finger flexion–extension PIP	0–100
0–90	Finger flexion–extension DIP	0–90
Full	Finger abduction	Full
Full	Finger adduction	Full

Abbreviations: DIP, distal interphalangeal; IP, interphalangeal; MP, metacarpophalangeal; PIP, proximal interphalangeal.

Table 2.3 Motor examination documentation

Left	Strength	Right
5/5	Elbow flexion	5/5
5/5	Elbow extension	5/5
5/5	Wrist flexion	5/5
5/5	Wrist extension	5/5
5/5	MP extension	5/5
5/5	Opposition pinch	5/5
5/5	Finger abduction	5/5

Abbreviation: MP, metacarpophalangeal.

References

[1] Dumanian GA, Segalman K, Buehner JW, Koontz CL, Hendrickson MF, Wilgis EF. Analysis of digital pulse-volume recordings with radial and ulnar artery compression. Plast Reconstr Surg. 1998; 102(6):1993–1998

[2] Thomson JC. Netter's Concise Orthopaedic Anatomy. 2nd ed. Philadelphia, PA: Saunders; 2010

[3] Rondinelli RD. Guides to the Evaluation of Permanent Impairment. 6th ed. Chicago, IL: American Medical Association; 2008

[4] Watson HK, Ashmead D, IV, Makhlouf MV. Examination of the scaphoid. J Hand Surg Am. 1988; 13(5): 657–660

[5] Kakinoki R. Examination of the upper extremity. In: Chang J, Neligan P, eds. Plastic Surgery: Volume 6: Hand and Upper Extremity Surgery. 4th ed. London: Elsevier; 2017:49–70

3 Radiographic Anatomy

Molly Vora and Laura Lewallen

Abstract

This chapter provides an overview of the pertinent musculoskeletal anatomy of the hand and wrist. Radiographic landmarks and descriptions of various views are provided. Several common fracture patterns are introduced, with representative radiographic images.

Keywords: Radiographs, anatomy, hand, wrist, X-rays, bones, fractures, dorsal, palmar, oblique, lateral views

I. Bony Anatomy of the Hand

- See ▶ Fig. 3.1.

II. Radiograph Views

- Three view of the wrist should be obtained: Posteroanterior (PA), lateral, and oblique views (▶ Fig. 3.2).
- Posteroanterior (PA) view—obtained with wrist and elbow at shoulder height; the radius and the ulna are parallel (▶ Fig. 3.2a).
  - Able to see the extensor carpi ulnaris groove radial to the midportion of the ulnar styloid.

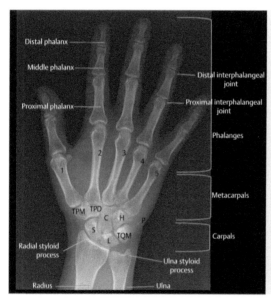

Fig. 3.1 Bony anatomy of the hand. C: Capitate; H: Hamate; L: Lunate; P: Pisiform; S: Scaphoid; TPD: Trapezoid; TPM: Trapezium; TQM: Triquetrum.

- Lateral view—obtained with elbow adducted to the side; shoulder, elbow, and wrist are in plane (▶ Fig. 3.2b).
  - Perpendicular to the PA view.
- Oblique view—hand is rotated externally 45 degrees from the PA position with fingers extended (▶ Fig. 3.2c).
  - Helpful in the trauma setting, including distal radius fractures, metacarpal fractures.

III. Joint Spaces: Parallelism and Symmetry

- The joint spaces of the wrist normally have a width of 2 mm or less (▶ Fig. 3.3).
  - Radiocarpal joint is slightly wider than the rest, carpometacarpal joints are slightly narrower.
  - The capitolunate joint is used as reference to which other joint spaces can be compared.

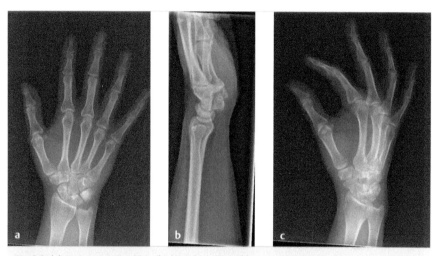

Fig. 3.2 (a) Posteroanterior (PA), (b) lateral, and (c) oblique views of the wrist.

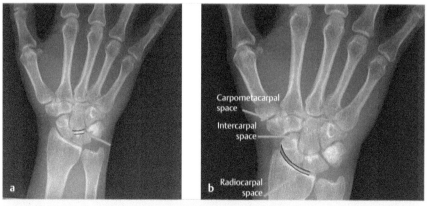

Fig. 3.3 (a) Joint spaces of the wrist. Arrow is pointing to capitolunate joint. (b) Observe the radiocarpal, intercarpal, and carpometacarpal joint spaces.

IV. Carpal Arcs

- Gilula's lines are three arcs drawn on the PA view, which are used to assess the alignment of the carpal bones (▶ Fig. 3.4):
  - First arc—smooth curve outlining the scaphoid, lunate, and triquetrum.
  - Second arc—the distal concave surfaces of the same bones.
  - Third arc—proximal curvature of the capitate and hamate.
  - Break in arc indicates fracture, ligamentous injury, and lunate/perilunate dislocation.

V. Shape of Carpal Bones

- Proximal row
  - Scaphoid: Shaped like a twisted peanut.
    - Largest bone in the proximal carpal row.
  - Lunate: Crescent-shaped
    - Normally trapezoidal in shape, but can appear triangular if displaced.
  - Triquetrum: Three-sided.
  - Pisiform: Pea-shaped.
- Distal row
  - Trapezium: Irregular-shaped four-sided.
  - Trapezoid: Four-sided
  - Capitate: Largest bone in the distal carpal row.
  - Hamate: Shaped like a hook.

VI. Wrist Analysis

- Ensure:
  - Adequate positioning of the patient's hand.
  - Normal alignment of the carpal bones.
  - No disruption of the three carpal arcs (disruption suggests ligament tear or fracture).
  - Proper shape and axis of the carpal bones (especially the scaphoid, lunate, and capitate).
  - Assess for fracture of the distal radius or carpal bones.

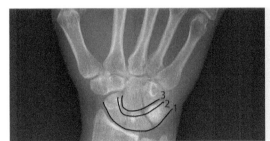

Fig. 3.4 Gilula's lines are three arcs drawn on the posteroanterior (PA) view. 1, first arc; 2, second arc; 3, third arc.

VII. Axis of the Carpal Bones

- Scaphoid axis
  - Line along the palmar aspect of the proximal and distal poles.
- Lunate axis (▶ Fig. 3.5)
  - Scapholunate angle: Perpendicular to the line along the palmar and dorsal aspects of the lunate.
    - Normal: 30–60.
- Capitate axis
  - Midportion of the proximal third metacarpal and proximal surface of the capitate.
  - Axis of rotation for all wrist motions passes through this carpal bone.
  - Capitolunate angle.
    - Abnormal: > 30 indicates instability.

VIII. Distal Radius Fracture

- Most common orthopaedic injury and accounts for 16% of all fractures.
- Frequently caused by a fall onto an outstretched hand (FOOSH).
- Diagnosis requires physical examination and standard wrist X-ray series.
- Degree of displacement and angulation is key factor.
  - Determines whether reduction and/or surgical intervention is necessary.
- Measurements include radial height (averaging between 10 and 13 mm), radial inclination (between 21 and 25 degrees), and volar tilt measured on a lateral radiograph (normal is ~10 degrees volar tilt; although acceptable range is dorsal angulation <5 degrees or within 20 degrees of contralateral distal radius; see ▶ Fig. 3.6).

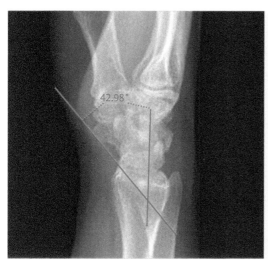

Fig. 3.5 The scapholunate angle is the angle between the long axis of the scaphoid (line along palmar aspect of the proximal to distal pole of the scaphoid) and the mid axis of the lunate (perpendicular to line along palmar and dorsal aspects of the lunate) on sagittal imaging of the wrist.

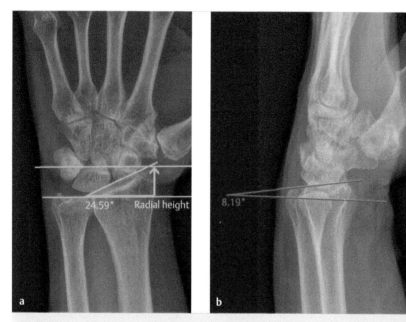

Fig. 3.6 Measurements shown on a standard X-ray. **(a)** Radial height and inclination and **(b)** volar tilt.

- Fracture types (eponyms):
  - Colles' fracture: Dorsally displaced, extra-articular fracture.
  - Smith's fracture: Volarly displaced, extra-articular fracture.
  - Barton's fracture: Intra-articular fracture of the distal radius with dislocation of the radiocarpal joint.
  - Chauffeur's fracture: Fracture of the radial styloid process.

IX. Ulnar Variance

- Length of the ulna compared to radius.
- Difference between ulnar and radial length should be <1 mm.
- Measured on PA radiographs with shoulder abducted 90 degrees, elbow flexed 90 degrees, and neutral forearm rotation (▸ Fig. 3.7).
  - Draw one line tangential to the articular surface of the ulna and perpendicular to its shaft, and another line tangential to the lunate fossa of the radius and perpendicular to its shaft.
  - Measure distance between these two lines (normal is 0–1 mm).
  - If ulna is longer than the radius = positive ulnar variance (UV) (may be associated with ulnar impaction syndrome).
  - If ulna is shorter than the radius = negative UV (may be associated with Kienbock's disease).

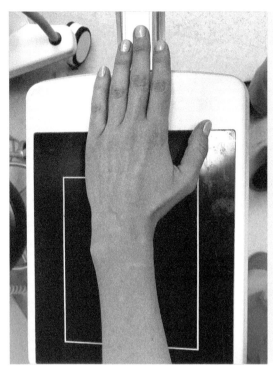

Fig. 3.7 Example of arm positioning for a standard PA radiograph.

X. Wrist Trauma

- Scaphoid fracture
  - Scaphoid is the most frequently fractured carpal bone (▶ Fig. 3.8).
- Recommended views
  - Scaphoid view (▶ Fig. 3.9).
    - 30-degree wrist extension, 20-degree ulnar deviation.
- Lunate dislocation (perilunate dissociation)
  - AP: Break in Gilula's arc, lunate and capitate overlap, lunate appears triangular (▶ Fig. 3.10a).
  - Lateral: Loss of colinearity of radius, lunate, and capitate, SL angle >70 degrees (▶ Fig. 3.10b).
- Hook of hamate fracture
  - 2% of carpal fractures.
  - The hook of hamate forms part of Guyon's canal.
  - The fracture is best seen on the carpal tunnel view.
  - CT scan if concern and not seen on plain X-ray (▶ Fig. 3.11).

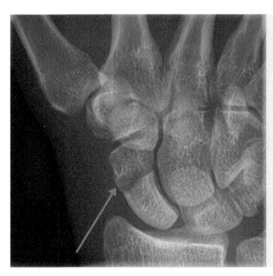

Fig. 3.8 Scaphoid fracture (*arrow*).

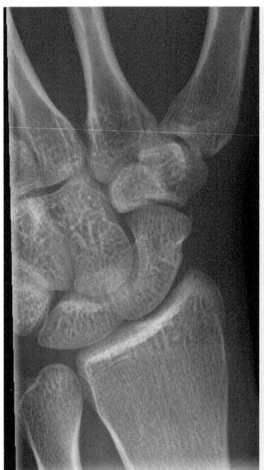

Fig. 3.9 Image shows a scaphoid view X-ray.

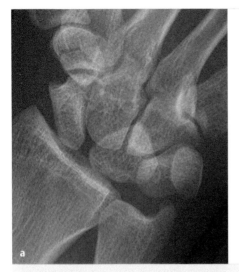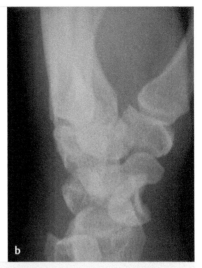

Fig. 3.10 Lunate dislocation (perilunate dissociation). **(a)** Anteroposterior (AP) and **(b)** lateral views.

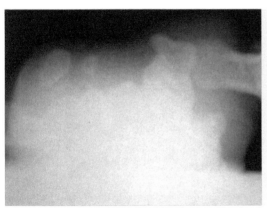

Fig. 3.11 CT scan showing hook of hamate fracture.

XI. Pediatric Hand Radiology

A. Skeletal Maturity

- A standard PA view of the hand and wrist (▶ Fig. 3.12).
- Physes (growth plates) are areas of developing cartilage at the ends of long bones, which ossify by skeletal maturity.
- The ulna and radius have growth plates at both ends, while metacarpals and phalanges have growth plates at only one end.
- Bone age can be used to predict remaining growth, approximate time a child will enter puberty, and a child's final height.

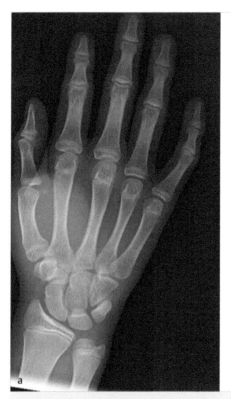 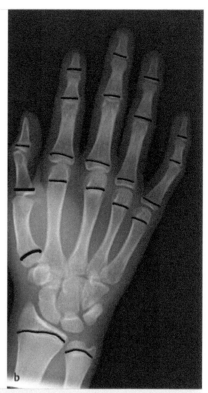

Fig. 3.12 (a, b) Posteroanterior (PA) view X-ray of a 13-year-old male showing location of the physes.

- Different methods to determine bone age by visualization of hand and wrist bones include: The Greulich & Pyle (GP) atlas, Tanner-Whitehouse (TW2) method, Gilsanz & Ratibin (GR) atlas, and automatic skeletal bone age assessment.

B. Pediatric Fractures

- Physeal injuries are common, as cartilage in children is weaker than surrounding ligaments.
- Salter-Harris classification (▶ Fig. 3.13).
  - Type I
    - 5–7%.
    - Fracture plane passes entirely through the growth plate.
  - Type II
    - 75% (most common).
    - Fracture passes through a portion of the growth plate and through the metaphysis.
  - Type III
    - 7–10%.
    - Fracture plane passes through some of the growth plate and down through the epiphysis.

○ Type IV
  – 10%.
  – Fracture plane passes directly through metaphysis, growth plate, and epiphysis.
○ Type V
  – < 1%.
  – Crushing type injury that causes damage to the growth plate by direct compression.
• Seymour's fracture
  ○ Fracture of the distal phalangeal physis and associated nail bed injury.
  ○ Often visualized on the lateral view X-ray (▶ Fig. 3.14).
  ○ Treatment typically includes: Nail plate removal, irrigation, reduction, nail bed repair, and antibiotics. In some cases open reduction and pinning of the DIP joint is indicated.

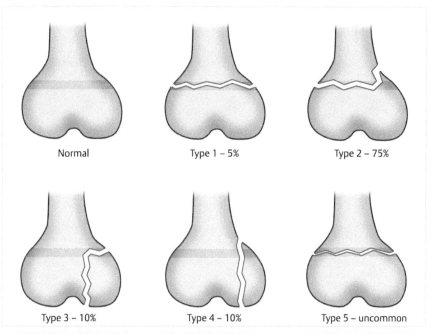

Fig. 3.13 Salter-Harris classification. Types I to V.

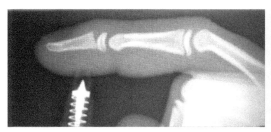

Fig. 3.14 Seymour's fracture.

4 Advanced Imaging

Laura M. Fayad and Jonathan Samet

Abstract

This chapter will explain when and why certain radiologic tests should be ordered for orthopaedic conditions of the wrist. Examples of multiple common orthopedic wrist entities will be discussed and shown.

Keywords: Wrist MRI, CT, scaphoid fracture, ganglion cyst, arthritis

I. Computed Tomography (CT)

- Advantages:
  - Excellent for bone detail.
  - Identifies small bone fragments better than MRI.
  - Identify fracture lines.
  - Can identify bone matrix of lesions better than MRI.
  - Can identify sclerosis and calcification better than MRI.
  - Very fast (seconds), much faster than MRI (wrist MRI 25–30 minutes).
  - Can image with metal hardware in place.
- Disadvantages:
  - Radiation exposure: Lower dose in extremities however.
  - Cannot see bone marrow edema.
  - Tendon evaluation limited.
  - Ligament evaluation poor.
  - Soft tissue evaluation limited.

II. MRI

- Advantages:
  - Excellent soft tissue detail.
  - Excellent for tendon and ligament evaluation.
  - Very sensitive for fluid (bone marrow edema, effusion, tenosynovitis).
  - Very sensitive for occult fracture (useful after negative X-ray).
  - Excellent to characterize soft tissue masses (fat, cyst, solid mass etc.).
- Disadvantages:
  - Images can be degraded by motion artifact.
  - Difficult to image with orthopedic metal hardware due to MRI artifact.
  - Much longer scanner times than CT.
  - Calcification and small bone fragments are hard to visualize.

III. Wrist Trauma

- Bone marrow edema
  - T2 hyperintense.

- T2 hyperintensity is accentuated with T2 fat suppression (T2 fat suppression, short tau inversion recovery [STIR]).
    - T1 hypointensity.
- Fracture
    - Acute
        - Fracture lines are linear and T1 hypointense.
        - On T2, fracture lines can be T2 hypointense or T2 hyperintense depending on if there is fluid in the fracture cleft or not.
    - Chronic (unhealed)
        - Fracture lines persist.
        - Sclerotic margins are hypointense on T1 and T2.
        - Persistent bone marrow edema.
        - Small cyst formation along fracture margin.
    - Scaphoid waist fracture (▶ Fig. 4.1)
        - Acute or chronic fracture line as above.
        - Significant bone marrow edema around the fracture line.
- Overuse injury and others
    - Physeal stress injuries in skeletally immature.
    - Physis is T2 slightly hyperintense and T1 hypointense.
    - Can request optional three-dimensional cartilage sequence for better evaluation.
    - Physis becomes thickened and irregular.
    - Classic example is "gymnast's wrist" (▶ Fig. 4.2).
- Extensor carpi ulnaris (ECU) tendinopathy
    - Common cause of ulnar sided pain.
    - Tendinosis is T2 hyperintense (grayish), unlike normal black tendon signal (▶ Fig. 4.3).
    - Partial tears will have T2 hyperintense (white) fluid clefts.
    - Can have associated tenosynovitis—T2 hyperintense fluid rim around ECU.

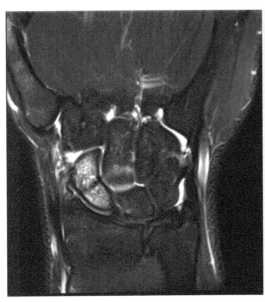

Fig. 4.1 Coronal T2 fat suppressed MRI image of the wrist shows T2 hyperintense signal compatible with bone marrow edema through the scaphoid bone. There is T2 hypointense fracture line through the scaphoid waist.

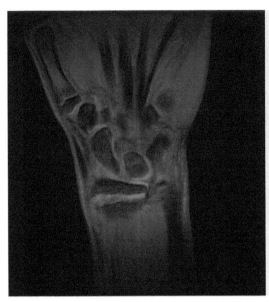

Fig. 4.2 Coronal three-dimensional spoiled gradient-recalled (3D SPGR) cartilage sequence of the wrist in a 12-year-old gymnast demonstrating thickening of the physis as seen in chronic physeal stress injury "gymnast's wrist."

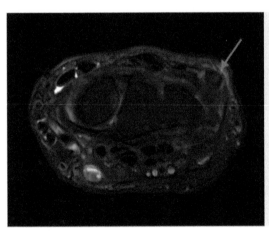

Fig. 4.3 Axial T2 fat suppressed wrist MRI showing mildly T2 hyperintense signal in the extensor carpi ulnaris (ECU) tendon compatible with tendinosis (*blue arrow*).

- Triangular fibrocartilage complex tear
  - Cause of ulnar sided pain.
  - Triangular fibrocartilage disc is T2 hypointense (black).
  - Two distal attachments to ulna—fovial and styloid; can have some T2 grayish signal normally due to fibrovascularity.
  - T2 hyperintense fluid signal to diagnose tear (▶ Fig. 4.4).
- Scapholunate ligament tear
  - On X-ray and CT, can be seen as widening of scapholunate interval (▶ Fig. 4.5).
  - On MRI, T2 hyperintense (fluid bright) gap instead of expected T2 hypointense ligament.

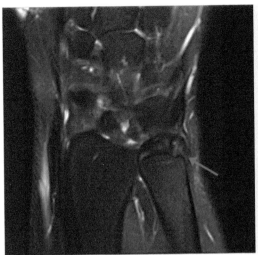

Fig. 4.4 Coronal T2 fat suppressed MRI image showing a partial tear (*blue arrow*) of the ulnar styloid attachment of the triangular fibrocartilage complex (TFCC).

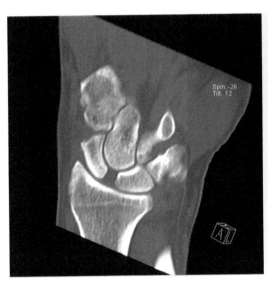

Fig. 4.5 Coronal CT reformatted image with significant widening of the scapholunate interval compatible with a tear of the scapholunate ligament.

IV. Inflammatory Arthritis MRI

- Joint effusion
  - ○ T2 hyperintense on fluid sensitive sequences (T2, PD).
- Synovitis
  - ○ T2 hyperintense (slightly less bright than fluid) (▶ Fig. 4.6a).
  - ○ On T1 post contrast, the synovium is hyperintense (enhancement) (▶ Fig. 4.6b).
- Erosions
  - ○ On T1 (without contrast), abnormal concavities/irregularities of the bone surfaces (▶ Fig. 4.6c).
  - ○ On T1 (with contrast), abnormal enhancing synovium extending into the erosions.

43

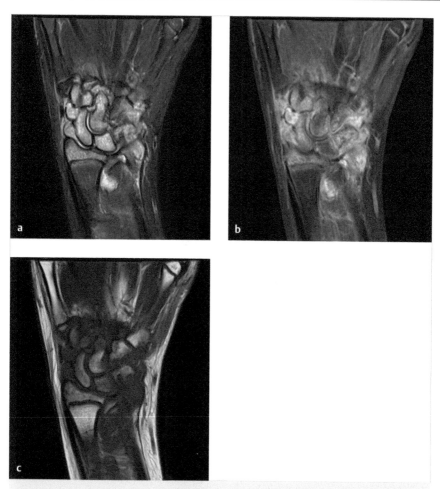

Fig. 4.6 (a) Coronal T2 fat suppressed, (b) coronal T1 fat suppressed post contrast, and (c) coronal T1 MRI images of the wrist. (a) Diffuse carpal bone marrow edema, (b) diffuse carpal bone marrow enhancement, and synovial hyperenhancement consistent with synovitis and inflammatory arthritis. (c) T1 hypointense concavities "bites" at multiple carpal bones representing erosions.

- Bone marrow edema
  ○ T2 hyperintense.
  ○ T2 hyperintensity is accentuated with T2 fat suppression (T2 fat suppression, STIR).
  ○ T1 hypointensity.

V. Neoplastic and Tumor-like Conditions

- Malignant soft tissue lesions (▶ Fig. 4.7a,b)
  ○ Rare.
  ○ T2 hyperintense, but noticeably less bright than fluid signal.
  ○ Solid or heterogenous enhancement on postcontrast.

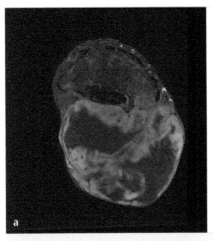 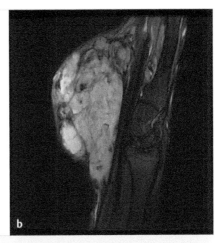

Fig. 4.7 **(a)** Axial T1 postcontrast fat suppressed and **(b)** sagittal T2 fat suppressed wrist MRI demonstrating a T2 hyperintense volar mass with heterogeneous postcontrast enhancement.

- Ganglion cyst
  - Very common cause of wrist "mass".
  - Typically dorsal over carpus.
  - T2 very hyperintense (similar to fluid signal) (▶ Fig. 4.8a–c).
  - Contrast is not usually needed.
  - Rim enhancement but no central solid enhancement on post contrast.

VI. Idiopathic

- Kienbock's disease
  - Avascular necrosis of the lunate.
  - Stage will determine appearance on imaging.
  - Initially normal on X-ray, will progress to sclerosis, collapse, and early osteoarthritis (▶ Fig. 4.9a,b).
  - On MRI, initially the lunate will be edematous, T2 hyperintense, and T1 hypointense (▶ Fig. 4.9b,c).
  - In more advanced stages, sclerosis will be T1 and T2 significantly hypointense (black).

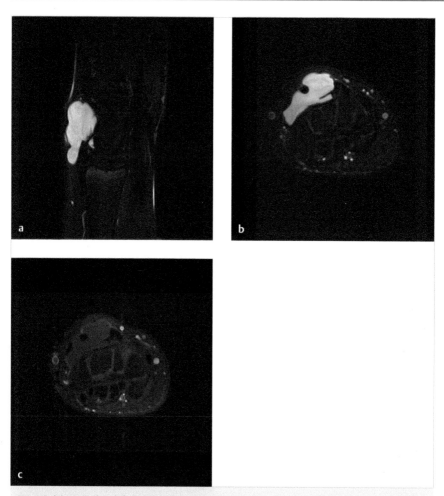

Fig. 4.8 (a) Sagittal and **(b)** axial T2 fat suppressed, and **(c)** axial T1 postcontrast fat suppressed images show a very T2 hyperintense lobulated dorsal wrist lesion. On post contrast that is minimal rim enhancement and no central enhancement, compatible with a ganglion cyst.

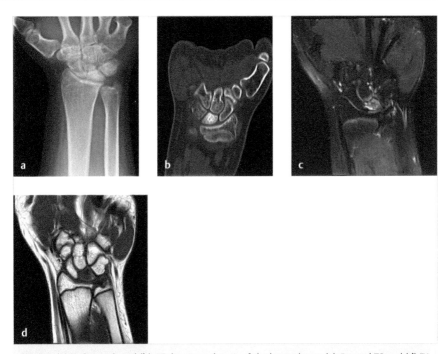

Fig. 4.9 (**a**) Radiograph and (**b**) CT showing sclerosis of the lunate bone. (**c**) Coronal T2 and (**d**) T1 fat suppressed MRI showing a T1 hypointense and T2 hyperintense lunate compatible with edema in early Kienbock's disease.

Suggested Readings

Capelastegui A, Astigarraga E, Fernandez-Canton G, Saralegui I, Larena JA, Merino A. Masses and pseudomasses of the hand and wrist: MR findings in 134 cases. Skeletal Radiol. 1999; 28(9):498–507

Cockenpot E, Lefebvre G, Demondion X, Chantelot C, Cotten A. Imaging of sports-related hand and wrist injuries: sports imaging series. Radiology. 2016; 279(3):674–692

Narváez JA, Narváez J, De Lama E, De Albert M. MR imaging of early rheumatoid arthritis. Radiographics. 2010; 30 (1):143–163, discussion 163–165

5 Electrodiagnostic Studies

Anthony F. Colon, Michael S. Shear, and Aviram M. Giladi

Abstract

The evaluation of neurologic or neuromuscular disorders through the application of electrophysiologic techniques, such as electromyography and nerve conduction studies, plays a pivotal role in the diagnosis and management of a wide array of pathologies. As an adjunct to a history and physical examination, electrodiagnostic studies aid in the physician's diagnostic approach. In this chapter, you will find an introduction to electrodiagnostic studies in the upper extremity, including analysis, interpretation, and common findings to aid in clinical practice.

Keywords: Electrodiagnostic, nerve conduction study, electromyography, neuropathy, upper extremity nerve compression

I. Anatomy

A. Anatomy of a Peripheral Nerve

- See ▶ Fig. 5.1.

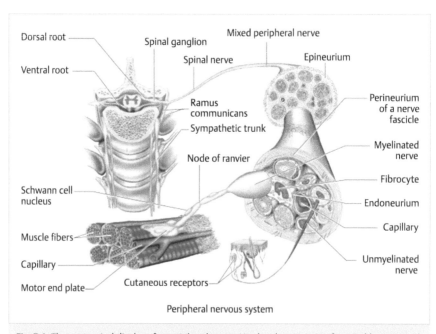

Fig. 5.1 The anatomical display of a peripheral nerve. Used with permission from Rohkamm R, ed. Color Atlas of Neurology. 2nd ed. Thieme; 2014.

B. Common Nerves Studied/Associated Lesions

- Upper trunk
  - Suprascapular nerve (C5–C6)
    - Compression can occur at suprascapular notch.
    - Weakness of supraspinatus and infraspinatus.
- Upper and middle trunk
  - Long thoracic nerve (C5–C7)
    - Compression/transection risk.
    - Weakness/loss of function of serratus anterior (loss of protraction and stabilization of scapula; causes scapular winging).
- Lateral cord
  - Musculocutaneous nerve (C5–C6)
    - Compression/entrapment by coracobrachialis (hypertrophy).
    - Weakness of coracobrachialis, biceps, and brachialis (flexion at elbow/glenohumeral joint, supination at radioulnar joint).
- Medial cord
  - Ulnar nerve (C8–T1)
    - Compression most commonly posterior to medial epicondyle of the elbow (cubital tunnel) or at Guyon's canal in the wrist.
    - Weakness, sensory loss, pain, and paresthesia in intrinsic muscles of hand and forearm flexors, and in the small and sometimes ring fingers (sensory).
- Lateral and medial cord
  - Median nerve (C5–T1)
    - Compression/entrapment at elbow (between heads of pronator teres) or more commonly the wrist (carpal tunnel).
    - Weakness, sensory loss, pain, and paresthesia in nerve distribution (anterior compartment of forearm, thenar muscle group, lumbricals, skin).
- Posterior cord
  - Axillary (C5–C6)
    - Trauma/stretch injury.
    - Weakness/loss of function of teres minor and deltoid muscle (loss of abduction by 15 to 90 degrees, flexion and extension of shoulder).
  - Radial nerve (C5–C6)
    - Compression or trauma (at risk with humeral fractures).
    - Weakness/loss of function/sensation in posterior compartment of arm and forearm (extension of elbow and wrist and fingers), sensory loss in dorsal hand.

II. Definitions

- Conduction velocity (CV)
  - The speed (meters/second) of an electrical impulse observed between two points.
- Latency (DL)
  - Onset latency
    - The amount of time (milliseconds) between stimulation and initiation of compound motor action potential.
  - Distal peak latency
    - The amount of time (milliseconds) between stimulation and peak waveform is observed in a sensory nerve action potential.

- Amplitude (Amp)
  - The difference in voltage observed between two points, proportional to the number and size of nerves depolarized.
- Duration
  - The time from onset of stimulus to termination.
- Compound muscle action potential (CMAP)
  - The muscle motor unit response to peripheral nerve stimulation, observed as a waveform.
- Sensory nerve action potential (SNAP)
  - The response of a sensory nerve following stimulation, observed as a waveform.

III. Physiology of Action Potential

The action potential of a nerve is dependent on the integrity of its components and electrical stimulation. The resting membrane potential of a muscle is affected by the concentration of sodium and potassium. Depolarization across the axonal membrane causes a stimulus at the neuromuscular junction, which in turn depolarizes skeletal muscle sarcolemma.

IV. Types of Studies

A. Electromyography

- The study of nerve and muscle integrity by observing electrical activity.
- Surface or intramuscular (needle) electrodes are used to stimulate and observe electrical activity that is produced by skeletal muscles. The placement of electrodes is dependent on the etiology.
  - Resting and insertional activity of the muscle is observed for comparison with voluntary muscle contraction.
    - Frequency, shape, and size of electrical impulses are observed. Various locations within muscle are studied to determine overall function.
    - Maximal voluntary contraction is used to correlate muscle function with electrical stimulation.
  - Motor unit action potential (MUAP) is the sum of electrical activity produced by stimulation. This is influenced by the number of motor units recruited. Factors affecting MUAP include fiber number, type, integrity, and metabolism.

B. Nerve Conduction Study

- It evaluates the ability for motor and sensory nerves to conduct electrical impulses to help determine the etiology and/or mechanism of symptoms. Determinants include the analysis of factors such as speed (conduction velocity), size (amplitude), and action potential shape. The stimulation and response recording by variously placed electrodes allow the clinician to analyze the integrity of motor and sensory components of the peripheral nervous system.

Nerve / Sites	Rec. site	Lat ms	Amp mV	Rel Amp %	Segments	Dist. cm	Vel m/s
R MEDIAN - APB							
Wrist	APB	3.55	10.6	100	Wrist - APB	8	
Elbow	APB	8.25	10.2	96.8	Elbow - wrist	24	51.1

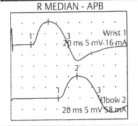

Fig. 5.2 Normal motor response of median nerve. Used with permission from the Curtis National Hand Center.

1. Electrophysiology

- Motor (▶ Fig. 5.2).
  - A peripheral nerve undergoes excitation by a stimulator and the muscle response is recorded by a separate electrode. In the upper extremity, the radial, ulnar, and median nerves are most commonly studied and evaluated.
    - The amount of time (milliseconds) between stimulation and initiation of compound motor action potential is designated as latency. An increase in latency is seen in loss of integrity or function of peripheral nerves by compression, demyelination, or other etiology.
  - The amplitude (mV) of a response, or the maximum size response of a generated action potential, can be compared between one or more muscle sites.
    - A decrease in amplitude can be seen in loss of muscle fiber recruitment, or from structural defects in the nerve or muscle itself.
  - The conduction velocity is the speed of an electrical impulse observed between two points. The velocity is calculated by stimulating multiple points along the same nerve, taking into account the distance and time it takes for an electrical impulse to propagate.
    - A decrease in conduction velocity can be observed if the structural integrity of the nerve, fascicles, axon, or myelination is compromised.
    - Conduction velocity = Distance (cm)/Time (ms).
- Sensory (▶ Fig. 5.3)
  - A peripheral nerve is stimulated with an electrical impulse and the observed response is recorded and analyzed. The observed response is the summation of all sensory action potentials, known as the SNAP.
    - Orthodromic—the nerve is stimulated distally and the action potential is recorded proximally (in the natural direction of the sensory response to the dorsal root ganglion and dorsal horn of the spinal cord).
    - Antidromic—the nerve is stimulated proximally and the action potential is recorded distally.

Nerve/Sites	Onset lat ms	Peak lat ms	NP Amp μV	PP Amp μV	Segments
R MEDIAN - Dig II antidromic					
1	2.80	3.45	14.0	23.0	1 - G1

R MEDIAN - Dig II antidromic

10 ms 20 μV. 16 mA

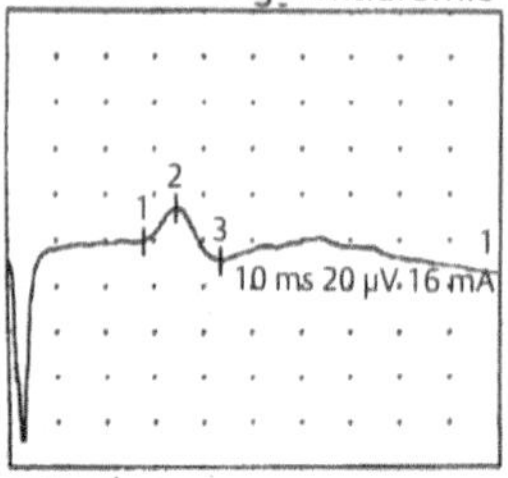

Fig. 5.3 Normal sensory response of median nerve. Used with permission from the Curtis National Hand Center.

- Parameters studied include latency (peak and onset), amplitude, duration of response, and conduction velocity. The number and size of activated sensory fibers affect the SNAP amplitude. The conduction velocity, duration, and latencies of stimulated sensory response are affected by internal and external components such as compression, transection, demyelination, and axonal injury.
- Common nerves studied in the upper extremity include the median and ulnar nerves.
- Mixed sensory and motor nerves are routinely evaluated, for example, in evaluating for carpal tunnel syndrome (CTS). The comparison of latencies and conduction velocities along different areas of the nerve provide information about the specific area of injury.
- H-reflex
  - Orthodromic evaluation of sensory and motor true reflex arc
    - Afferent loop includes type 1a sensory fibers to dorsal root ganglion and dorsal horn.
    - Efferent loop includes response from ventral horn and motor axons to produce muscle response.
    - Utility in assessing proximal damage to sensory or motor pathways, including radiculopathies or avulsions (especially cervical injuries).
- F-wave
  - Evaluation of motor nerve to identify structural integrity issues of proximal nerves such as radiculopathies and demyelinating disorders.
    - Supramaximal electrical impulse provided distally which travels from the peripheral motor nerve to the ventral horn and back down motor nerve distally.
    - High sensitivity in identifying demyelinating neuropathies due to proximal conduction slowing.

V. Limitations

A. Patient Limitations

- Temperature
  - Most important physiologic factor; upper extremity temperature ideally >33°; conduction velocity and distal latency are inaccurate in suboptimal conditions.
- Obesity
  - An increased distance between the surface of the skin and the muscle can alter study quality and accuracy.
- Peripheral vascular disease
  - Can affect results due to thickening of skin and skin breakdown.
- Wounds
  - Can limit surface area of examination as well as cause inaccurate results.

B. User Dependent

- Experience of the examiner and knowledge of potential injury etiologies are crucial in order to optimize the study.

VI. Normal Values

Literature review by the Normative Data Task Force helped to establish reference points for electrodiagnostic studies in the upper and lower extremities (▶ Table 5.1 and ▶ Table 5.2).

Table 5.1 Reference values for six major sensory nerve conduction studies in adults

Nerves	Size (N)	Amplitude: lower limit (third percentile) (µV)		Latency: upper limit (97th percentile) (ms)	
		Onset-to-peak	Peak-to-peak	Onset	Peak
Superficial radial sensory (antidromic, 10 cm)	212	7	11	2.2	2.8
Median sensory* (antidromic to second digit, wrist 14 cm, palm 7 cm)	258	11 (wrist)	13 (wrist)	3.3 (wrist)	4 (wrist)
Amplitude (wrist) by age and BMI**					
(19–49) BMI < 24		17	19		
(19–49) BMI ≥ 24		11	13		
(50–79) BMI < 24		9	15		
(50–79) BMI ≥ 24		7	8		
Ulnar sensory (antidromic to fifth digit, 14 cm)	258	10	9	3.1	4.0
Amplitude (wrist) by age and BMI**					
(19–49) BMI < 24		14	13		
(19–49) BMI ≥ 24		11	8		
(50–79) BMI < 24		10	13		
(50–79) BMI ≥ 24		5	4		
Medial antebrachial cutaneous sensory (antidromic, 10 cm)	207	4	3		2.6
Lateral antebrachial cutaneous sensory (antidromic, 10 cm)	213	5	6		2.5
Sural sensory (antidromic, 14 cm)	230	4	4	3.6	4.5

Note: BMIs calculated as: $BMI = W/H^2$, where W is the patient's weight (in kg) and H is the patient's height (in m).

* Median sensory NCS data shown where recorded at digit 2. Normative data recorded at digit 3 are also available in the same article.
The digit 3 findings are similar in magnitude to data derived from digit 2.
** The lower limits of onset-to-peak amplitudes are shown as mean−2 SD, showing the statistically significant effects of age and BMI on the amplitudes of the median and ulnar sensory nerves at the wrist (P < 0.01). Data sets normalized by square-root transformation.
Used with permission from the American Association of Neuromuscular & Electrodiagnostic Medicine.

Table 5.2 Reference values for four major motor nerve conduction studies in adults

Nerves	Size (N)	Distal amplitude (mV)		Conduction velocity (m/s)		Distal latency (ms)	
		Subgroups	Lower limit third %	Subgroups	Lower limit third %	Subgroups	Upper limit 97th %
Median motor	249	All ages	4.1*	All ages	49*	All ages	4.5*
		Amplitude by age		CV by age and gender		Distal latency by age and gender	
		19–39 y	5.9	19–39 y, men	49	19–49 y, men	4.6
		40–59 y	4.2	19–39 y, women	53	19–49 y, women	4.4
		60–79 y	3.8	40–79 y, men	47	50–79 y, men	4.7
				40–79 y, women	51	50–79 y, women	4.4
Ulnar motor	248	All ages	7.9*	Below elbow	52*	All ages	3.7*
				Across elbow	43*		
				Above elbow	50		
				CV drop across the elbow	15		
				CV drop across the elbow (%)	23		
Fibular (peroneal) motor	242	All ages	1.3*	CV ankle to below fibular head	38*	All ages	6.5*
				CV ankle to below fibular head by age and height			
				19–39 y, <170 cm	43		
				19–39 y, >170 cm	37		
				40–79 y, <170 cm	39		
				40–79 y, >170 cm	36		
		Amplitude by age					
		19–39 y	2.6	CV across fibular head	42*		
		40–79 y	1.1	CV drop across the fibular head	6*		

Table 5.2 *(Continued)* Reference values for four major motor nerve conduction studies in adults

Nerves	Size (N)	Distal amplitude (mV)		Conduction velocity (m/s)		Distal latency (ms)	
		Subgroups	Lower limit third %	Subgroups	Lower limit third %	Subgroups	Upper limit 97th %
		% drop in amplitude from ankle to below fibula	32%*				
		% drop in amplitude across fibular head	25%*	% drop in CV across fibular head	12%*		
Tibial motor	250	All ages	4.4*	All ages	39*	All ages	6.1*
		Amplitude by age		CV by age and height			
		19–29 y		19–49 y, <160 cm	44		
		30–59 y		19–49 y, <160–170 cm	42		
		60–79 y		19–49 y, ≥170 cm	37		
		Amplitude drop from ankle to knee	10.3*	50–79 y, <160 cm	40		
		% drop in amplitude from ankle to knee	71%*	50–79 y, <160–170 cm	37		
				50–79 y, ≥170 cm	34		

* Values for the entire sample for each nerve encompassing all ages.
Used with permission from the American Association of Neuromuscular & Electrodiagnostic Medicine.

Suggested Readings

Chen S, Andary M, Buschbacher R, et al. Electrodiagnostic reference values for upper and lower limb nerve conduction studies in adult populations. Muscle Nerve. 2016; 54(3):371–377

Chichkova RI, Katzin L. EMG and nerve conduction studies in clinical practice. Pract Neurol. 2010:32–38

Eisen A, Fisher M. Recommendations for the Practice of Clinical Neurophysiology: The F Wave. Elsevier Science B.V.; 1999. http://www.clinph-journal.com/pb/assets/raw/Health Advance/journals/clinph/Chapter6–3.pdf. Accessed August 12, 2018

Hammert W, Boyer M, Bozentka D. ASSH Manual of Hand Surgery. Philadelphia: Wolters Kluwer Health; 2015:294–350

Kimura J. Electrodiagnosis in diseases of nerve and muscle. Oxford: Oxford University Press; 2013

Rana AQ, Ghouse AT, Govindarajan R. Nerve conduction studies. In: Neurophysiology in Clinical Practice. In Clinical Practice. Springer, Cham; 2017:59–62

Rohkamm R, ed. Color Atlas of Neurology. 1st ed. Thieme; 2004

Siao P, Cros D, Vucic S. Practical Approach to Electromyography. New York: Demos Medical; 2011

Warren SD. (2007). Manual of Nerve Conduction Study and Surface Anatomy for Needle Electromyography. 4th ed. Journal of Clinical Neuromuscular Disease. 8. 170. 10.1097/01.cnd.0000262745.42357.39

Wolfe S, Hotchkiss R, Pederson W, Kozin S, Cohen M. Green's Operative Hand Surgery. Philadelphia: Elsevier; 2017:979–1146

6 Fractures, Dislocations, and Ligament Injuries of the Hand

Richard Samade and Hisham Awan

Abstract

This chapter will provide the reader a concise overview of various traumatic injuries that are commonly encountered in the hand. The osseous structures of interest described in this section include the metacarpals and phalanges. For each pathology summarized, emphasis is placed on descriptions of the mechanism of injury, relevant anatomy, clinical presentation, appropriate imaging, and recommended treatments. Figures with radiographs are also provided to illustrate key pathologies and treatments. This chapter is designed to provide an easily readable reference that will aid the orthopaedic practitioner in determining appropriate treatment for a traumatic pathology encountered during consultations in the emergency department, inpatient ward, or outpatient clinic. Thus, it will ideally be a useful resource for orthopaedic residents, advanced practitioners, and practicing orthopedic surgeons. References for the core material outlined here are listed at the end of this chapter and contain further information on each topic presented for the interested reader.

Keywords: Trauma, fracture, dislocation, intra-articular, extra-articular, ligament, tear

I. Fractures of the Metacarpals

A. Thumb Metacarpal Base Fractures

- Mechanism of injury
  - Trauma (e.g., fall or punch) with axial loading and partial flexion of the thumb metacarpal.[1,2]
- Relevant anatomy and epidemiology
  - Fractures can be extra-articular, intra-articular with a stable volar-ulnar fragment (a Bennett's fracture), or intra-articular with comminution (a Rolando's fracture, see ▶ Fig. 6.1a).
  - Deforming forces: Adductor pollicis, abductor pollicis longus, and extensor pollicis longus.
- Clinical presentation
  - Pain, swelling, and limited range of motion (ROM) at the base of the thumb.
- Imaging used for diagnosis
  - Thumb X-ray series is best for diagnosis and to evaluate for intra-articular extension.
- Treatment
  - Nonoperative: Stable, extra-articular, and <30 degrees of angular deformity can be splinted.
  - Operative: If unstable or intra-articular, then proceed with open reduction internal fixation (ORIF) versus closed reduction percutaneous pinning (CRPP) (▶ Fig. 6.1b).

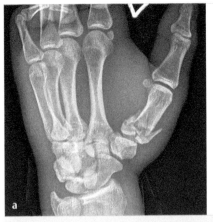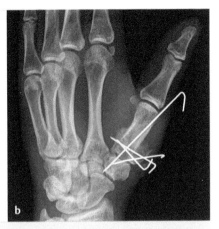

Fig. 6.1 (a) A lateral radiograph of a hand with a comminuted intra-articular base of thumb fracture (Rolando variant) with associated soft tissue swelling. **(b)** Rolando's fracture shown in **(a)** after open reduction and percutaneous pinning.

B. Metacarpal Base Fractures Other than the Thumb

- Mechanism of injury
  - Direct trauma (e.g., from punch) is the mechanism of all non-thumb metacarpal fractures.[1,2,3,4]
- Relevant anatomy and epidemiology
  - May be extra-articular or intra-articular, usually apex dorsal due to intrinsic forces.
  - It is important to evaluate for concomitant carpometacarpal (CMC) joint dislocation.
- Clinical presentation
  - Pain and swelling in middle hand present, sometimes with open wounds or tenting of skin.
  - Evaluate all metacarpal fractures for malrotation by confirming that the cascade of fingertips, when the patient makes a closed fist, points to the scaphoid.
- Imaging used for diagnosis
  - Usually, a full hand X-ray series suffices to diagnose all metacarpal fractures.
- Treatment
  - Nonoperative: Treat with reduction and splinting in intrinsic plus position for:
    - A nondisplaced intra-articular fracture.
    - An extra-articular fracture with no malrotation and with acceptable angulation (10 degrees for index [IF], 20 degrees for long [LF], 30 degrees for ring [RF], and 40 degrees for small [SF] fingers).
  - Operative: If none of the above, consider proceeding to ORIF with plate versus CRPP.

C. Metacarpal Shaft Fractures

- Relevant anatomy and epidemiology
  - Fractures may have transverse or oblique orientation, with the latter prone to shortening.[1,2,3,4]

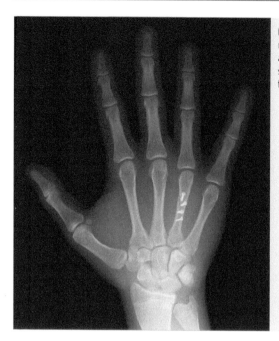

Fig. 6.2 An anteroposterior (AP) radiograph of a hand demonstrating an unstable oblique metacarpal shaft fracture of the ray of the ring finger, stabilized with four screws.

- Treatment
  - Nonoperative: Can do closed reduction and immobilization if no malrotation and acceptable angulation (10 degrees for IF, 20 degrees for LF, 30 degrees for RF, and 40 degrees for SF).
  - Operative: Consider ORIF with plate/screws versus CRPP for oblique fractures (▶ Fig. 6.2).

D. Metacarpal Head and Neck Fractures

- Relevant anatomy and epidemiology
  - Head fractures commonly lead to joint incongruity if displaced or comminuted.[1,2,3,4]
- Treatment
  - Nonoperative: Can be treated with reduction and splinting in intrinsic plus position for nondisplaced intra-articular head or extra-articular neck fractures (with no malrotation and acceptable angulation of 10–15 degrees for IF and LF, up to 40 degrees for RF, and up to 60 degrees for SF).
  - Operative: If none of the above, consider ORIF with plate/screws versus CRPP versus head arthroplasty (if a high degree of comminution is present).

II. Fractures of the Phalanges

A. Proximal Phalangeal Fractures

- Mechanism of injury
  - Trauma with axial loading or crushing is the typical insult for all phalangeal fractures.[1,2,3,5]

- Relevant anatomy and epidemiology
  - May involve the shaft, neck, or condyles, with an intrinsic deforming force.
- Clinical presentation
  - Must evaluate for concomitant dislocation and entrapped volar plate needing removal.
  - Also, one must evaluate for angulation, malrotation, shortening, and stability.
- Imaging used for diagnosis
  - An X-ray series specific to the affected finger should be used for all phalangeal fractures.
- Treatment
  - Nonoperative: Stable and nondisplaced shaft and neck fractures can be splinted (angulation <10 degrees, no malrotation, stable after reduction, and <2 mm of shortening).
  - Operative: All condyle and unstable neck/shaft fractures undergo ORIF versus CRPP (▶ Fig. 6.3).

B. Middle Phalangeal Fractures

- Relevant anatomy and epidemiology
  - Can involve the shaft or base (in a fracture–dislocation) and flexor digitorum superficialis (FDS) is a deforming force.[1,2,3,5]
- Clinical presentation
  - Must evaluate for concomitant dislocation and entrapped volar plate needing removal.
- Treatment
  - Nonoperative: Shaft fractures (buddy taping, if <10 degrees angulation and no malrotation).
  - Operative: ORIF versus CRPP if displaced/unstable, especially intra-articular (▶ Fig. 6.4).

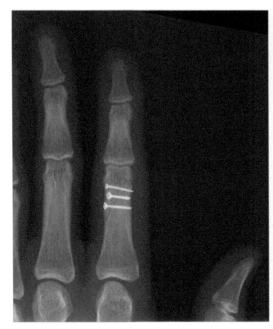

Fig. 6.3 An anteroposterior (AP) radiograph of the index finger proximal phalanx demonstrating lag screw fixation of an unstable oblique shaft fracture.

C. Distal Phalangeal Fractures

- Relevant anatomy and epidemiology
  - May manifest with tuft, shaft, dorsal intra-articular (mallet finger), or volar intra-articular (jersey finger) fracture patterns.[1,2]
- Clinical presentation
  - If a subungal hematoma exists, consider evacuation and evaluation for nail bed injury.
  - A nail bed injury is indicative of an open fracture when the distal phalanx is injured.
- Treatment
  - Nonoperative: Splint if stable without displacement, repair nail bed with absorbable suture.
  - Operative: Usually CRPP versus ORIF for jersey fingers and unstable mallet fingers.

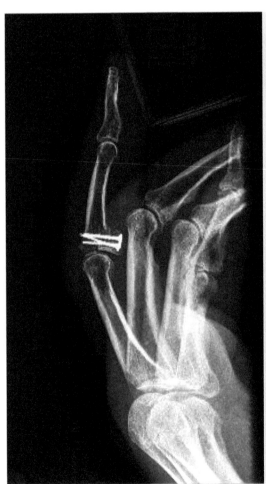

Fig. 6.4 A lateral radiograph of the ring finger demonstrating the use of a hemihamate autograft for addressing an unstable intra-articular base of middle phalanx fracture.

III. Dislocations of the Carpometacarpal, Metacarpophalangeal, and Interphalangeal Joints

A. Carpometacarpal Joint (CMCJ) Dislocations

- Mechanism of injury
  - Direct traumatic force in the direction of dislocation (dorsal is more common than volar).[1]
- Relevant anatomy and epidemiology
  - More commonly involves the thumb CMCJ due to hypermobility.
- Clinical presentation
  - Pain, deformity, and lack of ROM at the base of the metacarpal.
- Imaging used for diagnosis
  - Obtain thumb X-ray series for thumb CMCJ dislocation and hand series for other CMCJs.
- Treatment
  - Nonoperative: Can be treated with blocking splint if stable closed reduction achieved.
  - Operative: Unstable or chronic dislocations treated with open versus closed reduction and percutaneous pinning (▶ Fig. 6.5).

B. Metacarpophalangeal Joint (MCPJ) Dislocations

- Relevant anatomy and epidemiology[1,2,3]
  - Juncturae tendinae and volar plate may become interposed and block reduction attempts.
- Clinical presentation
  - Pain, deformity, and lack of ROM at the base of the proximal phalanx.

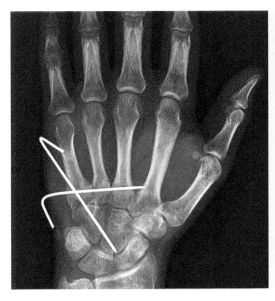

Fig. 6.5 An anteroposterior (AP) radiograph of the hand after open reduction and Kirschner wire fixation of chronic dislocations of the ring and small finger carpometacarpal (CMC) joints.

- Imaging used for diagnosis
  - Obtain X-rays of the affected finger to evaluate MCPJ and interphalangeal joints (IPJs).
- Treatment
  - Nonoperative: After successful closed reduction, place splint blocking direction of dislocation.
  - Operative: Irreducible dislocations require open reduction via dorsal or volar approach.

C. Proximal Interphalangeal Joint (PIPJ) Dislocations

- Relevant anatomy and epidemiology[1,2,3,6]
  - Volar plate interposition (dorsal dislocations) and central slip injury (volar dislocations) may be associated with these injuries.
  - Rotatory dislocations occur with the P1 condyle between the central slip and lateral band.
- Clinical presentation
  - Pain, deformity, and lack of ROM at the base of the middle phalanx (▶ Fig. 6.6).
- Imaging used for diagnosis
  - Obtain X-rays of the affected finger to evaluate MCPJ and the IPJs.
- Treatment
  - Nonoperative: After successful closed reduction, place splint blocking direction of dislocation.
  - Operative: For irreducible dislocations and repair of central slip injuries, if present.

D. Distal Interphalangeal Joint (DIPJ) Dislocations

- Relevant anatomy and epidemiology.[1,2,3,6]

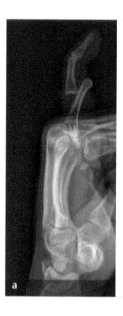
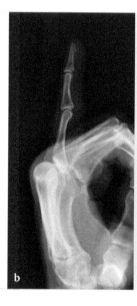

Fig. 6.6 (a) A lateral radiograph of the small finger demonstrating an open dorsal proximal interphalangeal (PIP) joint dislocation. (b) A lateral radiograph of the small finger PIP joint of the patient depicted in (a), following reduction, irrigation, debridement, wound closure, antibiotics, and splinting.

- Flexor digitorum profundus (FDP) and volar plate may become interposed and block reduction attempts.
- Clinical presentation
  - Pain, deformity, and lack of ROM at the base of the distal phalanx.
- Imaging used for diagnosis
  - Obtain X-rays of the affected finger to evaluate MCPJ and the IPJs.
- Treatment
  - Usually with closed reduction/splinting, but interposed tissue requires open reduction.

IV. Common Hand Ligamentous Injuries

A. Thumb Ulnar Collateral (UCL) and Radial Collateral Ligament (RCL) Injuries

- Mechanism of injury[1,2]
  - Thumb UCL avulsions and tears, due to hyperextension or hyperabduction of the MCPJ, may be acute (e.g., skier's thumb) or chronic (e.g., gamekeeper's thumb).
  - Thumb RCL avulsions and tears are due to a hyperadduction injury of the MCPJ.
- Relevant anatomy and epidemiology
  - Both the UCL and RCL are composed of proper and accessory collateral ligaments.
  - A Stener lesion is adductor aponeurosis interposition between the UCL and MCPJ.
- Clinical presentation
  - Evaluate for >35 degrees opening or >20 degrees variability between hands with stress at 30 degrees of MCPJ flexion (assess proper ligament) and full MCPJ extension (assess accessory ligament).
- Imaging used for diagnosis
  - Obtain X-rays of the affected thumb for initial evaluation and follow-up (▶ Fig. 6.7).
  - MRI may be used for confirmation with equivocal history and examination (▶ Fig. 6.8).
- Treatment
  - Nonoperative: Thumb spica splint and therapy for acute partial and chronic tears.
  - Operative: Repair (for acute tears) or reconstruction (for chronic tears), using suture anchors.

B. Sagittal Band (SB) Injuries

- Mechanism of injury
  - Frequently due to direct trauma to the MCPJ (e.g., patient punches with closed fist).[1,7]
- Relevant anatomy and epidemiology
  - The radial SB is more frequently injured compared to the ulnar SB.
- Clinical presentation
  - MCPJ flexion leads to subluxation of the extensor tendon opposite to the injured band.
  - Evaluate for other injuries (e.g. central slip rupture with boutonnierre deformity).
- Imaging used for diagnosis
  - X-rays and MRI of the hand can help establish the location and extent of SB tears.
- Treatment
  - Nonoperative: Extension splinting for acute SB tears.
  - Operative: Direct repair versus extensor tendon centralization for chronic SB tears.

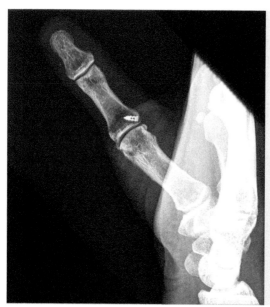

Fig. 6.7 A postoperative anteroposterior (AP) radiograph of the right thumb demonstrating 2.7 mm suture anchor fixation for repair of a thumb ulnar collateral (UCL) tear.

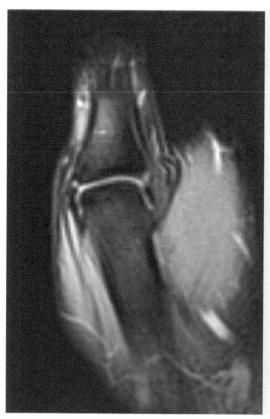

Fig. 6.8 A coronal series in a T2-weighted, fat-suppressed MRI sequence of the right thumb, demonstrating disruption of the proper collateral ligament of the thumb radial collateral ligament (RCL).

References

[1] Wolfe S, Pederson W, Hotchkiss R, Kozen S, eds. Green's Operative Hand Surgery. 6th ed. Philadelphia, PA: Churchill Livingstone; 2010

[2] Eltorai A, Eberson C, Daniels A, eds. Orthopedic Surgery Clerkship: A Quick Reference Guide for Senior Medical Students. New York, NY: Springer International AG; 2017

[3] Baltera R, Hastings H. Fractures and dislocations: hand. In: Hammert WC, ed. ASSH Manual of Hand Surgery. Philadelphia, PA: Lippincott Williams and Wilkins; 2010

[4] Wong VW, Higgins JP. Evidence-based medicine: management of metacarpal fractures. Plast Reconstr Surg. 2017; 140(1):140e–151e

[5] Verver D, Timmermans L, Klaassen RA, van der Vlies CH, Vos DI, Schep NWL. Treatment of extra-articular proximal and middle phalangeal fractures of the hand: a systematic review. Strateg Trauma Limb Reconstr. 2017; 12(2):63–76

[6] Shah CM, Sommerkamp TG. Fracture dislocation of the finger joints. J Hand Surg Am. 2014; 39(4):792–802

[7] Grandizio LC, Klena JC. Sagittal band, boutonniere, and pulley injuries in the athlete. Curr Rev Musculoskelet Med. 2017; 10(1):17–22

7 Carpal Fractures and Dislocations

Kevin O'Malley, Jay L. Mottla, and Michael W. Kessler

Abstract
Carpal fractures and dislocations are rare injuries, with injury to the scaphoid comprising the majority. Evaluation of patients with suspected carpal injuries begins with thorough history taking as well as detailed physical diagnosis. To correctly diagnose and treat injuries of the carpus a comprehensive understanding of the unique anatomical features, complex interactions between the bones and ligaments, and specific radiological assessments is required. For timely and proper treatment the evaluator must always have a high index of suspicion for these injuries.

Keywords: Carpus fractures, scaphoid fractures, perilunate instability, triquetrum fractures, trapezium fractures, capitate fractures, hamate fractures

I. Scaphoid

A. Background

- Most common carpal fracture (60%).
- Demographics: Young men 15 to 25 years of age.
- Risk factors include college football players, military personal, and low socioeconomic class.
- Mechanism
  - Fall onto hyperextended wrist (>95 degrees extension).
    - Excessive stress at scaphoid waist.

B. Presentation

1. Physical Examination

- Tenderness at anatomic snuff box, longitudinal thumb compression, scaphoid tubercle, painful ulnar deviation, and decreased grip strength.
  - Snuff box tenderness has high sensitivity but low specificity.
  - Combination of maneuvers is recommended to increase specificity and sensitivity.

C. Evaluation

1. Imaging

- Radiographs
  - Standard series (four views): Posteroanterior (PA), lateral, and oblique hand radiographs; scaphoid view radiograph; PA wrist with ulnar deviation (only about 64% sensitive).
  - If negative on imaging, commonly treated with 2 weeks of thumb spica cast immobilization followed by repeat radiograph.
  - Overtreat five out of six patients with suspected injuries.
  - Will miss 9% of scaphoid fractures.

- Computed tomography (CT)
  - Sensitivity = 0.71
  - Specificity = 0.99
- Magnetic resonance imaging (MRI)
  - Most utilized advanced imaging in North America
    - Sensitivity = 0.88
    - Specificity = 0.99
- Bone scintigraphy
  - Highest diagnostic accuracy
    - Sensitivity = 0.99
    - Specificity = 0.86
  - Highest radiation exposure
  - Diagnostic delay of 72 hours

D. Classification

- Many classification systems available, all with varying limitations and clinical utility.
  - At least 13 based on fracture location/orientation/stability/displacement.
- Limitation of classifications
  - Many rely on radiographs with limited sensitivity and potential underestimation of displacement.
  - Poor intraobserver reliability.
  - Most have poor prediction of fracture union.
- Specific classifications
  - Herbert
    - Stable: Tubercle fractures and incomplete waist fractures.
    - Unstable: Complete distal oblique fractures, complete waist fractures, proximal pole fractures, and transscaphoid perilunate fracture-dislocations.
  - Mayo
    - Location: Distal tubercle, distal intra-articular surface, distal third, waist, and proximal pole.
  - Rousse
    - Orientation: Transverse, horizontal oblique, and vertical oblique (highest rates of nonunion and increased shear stress).

E. Management

- Treatment algorithms must be personalized and depend on many variables:
  - Fracture location.
  - Fracture displacement.
  - Patient-specific factors.

1. Nondisplaced Scaphoid Waist

- Nonoperative: Short arm cast with or without thumb immobilization for 6 weeks. Then obtain CT scan of wrist. If CT scan demonstrates healing, transition to wrist brace for another 4 to 6 weeks.
  - Union expected from 2 to 3 months.

- Operative
  - Percutaneous treatment
    - Recent literature has shown faster time to union with lower complication rate than nonoperative management.
    - Variables affecting patient's decision-making for operative versus nonoperative management are out-of-pocket cost and surgical apprehension.

2. Proximal Pole Fractures and Unstable Scaphoid Fractures

- Operative management generally recommended
  - Unstable fractures are defined by over 1 mm of displacement, comminution, associated perilunate fracture-dislocation, intra-scaphoid angle of over 35 degrees, scapholunate angle of over 60 degrees, or radiolunate angle of over 15 degrees.
- Goals of operative fixation
  - Rigid fixation for primary bone healing.
- Approaches for operative fixation
  - A meta-analysis comparing volar and dorsal approaches for acute scaphoid fractures showed no difference in union rates, functional outcomes, or pain.
  - Volar approach: It divides the radial extrinsic carpal ligaments. It may result in scaphotrapeziotrapezoid (STT) arthritis. There is an increased rate of ulnar deviation with the volar approach, but this is of uncertain clinical significance.
  - Dorsal approach: It provides more consistent central screw position, but places the scaphoid blood supply and extensor tendons at risk.
  - Percutaneous.

3. Methods of Fixation

- Cannulated Herbert screw
  - Benefits: Improved union rate, improved return to work, and improved functional outcomes.
  - Technique
    - Screws should be within the central one-third axis of the scaphoid utilizing the longest screw possible that is ideally perpendicular to the fracture.
    - Central placement with longer screws will provide greater stiffness, a reduction of forces at the fracture site, and a reduction in time to union.
    - Anatomic studies show safe screw lengths of 27 mm in men and 23 mm in women.
    - Arthroscopic-assisted reduction can assist in determining screw length by providing direct visual joint visualization.
- Other
  - K-wires, staples, plate fixation.
    - Plate fixation may be indicated in osteoporotic fractures.

F. Complications

1. Most Common

- Delayed union (time to union >6 months).
- Nonunion
  - Delayed diagnosis and treatment increases the risk for nonunion and may occur in 5 to 25% of cases.

- Post-traumatic arthritis.
- Malunion
  ○ Amadio et al (1989) reported patients with lateral intrascaphoid angle of over 45 degrees had unsatisfactory outcomes in 73% of cases and post-traumatic arthritis in 54% compared to 17% unsatisfactory outcomes without malunion.
- Tendon rupture.
- Complex regional pain syndrome (CRPS).
- Osteonecrosis
  ○ Osteonecrosis is seen in 13 to 50% of scaphoid fractures with higher rates seen in proximal pole fractures.
- Prominent hardware.

2. Complication Differences between Nonoperative and Operative Management

- In a recent systematic review of minimally and nondisplaced scaphoid fractures, there was no significant difference between operative treatment (14%) and nonoperative treatment (7%) in terms of complications.
  ○ The most common complications in the operative group were delayed union, nonunion, and hardware-related complications.
  ○ The most common complications in nonoperative group consisted of predominantly delayed union and nonunion complications.
  ○ Malunion occurs in both operatively and nonoperatively treated scaphoid fractures where the distal fragment flexes and the proximal fragment extends resulting in a humpback deformity.

II. Perilunate Instability

A. Background

- Perilunate dislocations and fracture-dislocations encompass a wide spectrum of injuries and typically result from high energy trauma.
  ○ Pure ligamentous perilunate dislocations are referred to as lesser arc injuries while greater arc injuries involve fractures most frequently of the scaphoid.
  ○ Mayfield et al (1980) described progressive perilunate instability in four stages:
    – Stage 1: Hyperextension of the carpal row with failure of the scapholunate ligament as the scaphoid extends beyond the limits of the lunate.
    – Stage 2: Dorsal dislocation of the scaphoid and distal carpal row from the lunate (perilunate dislocation).
    – Stage 3: The third stage occurs with continued hyperextension that now results in the fracture of the triquetrum or rupture of the lunotriquetral ligaments as the triquetrum extends.
    – Stage 4: Results from an intact radioscaphocapitate (RSC) ligament pushing the capitate proximally with the lunate then dislocating.
  ○ Herzberg et al (1993) further subclassified lunate dislocations based on lunate rotation:
    – Worsening results were seen with increasing lunate rotation and were attributed to higher energy mechanisms with increased ligament injury and soft tissue interposition.

B. Presentation

- Relatively limited physical examination findings beyond pain, decreased wrist range of motion, and possibly carpal tunnel related symptoms.
  - Diagnosis requires a high index of suspicion following high energy wrist trauma.

C. Evaluation

- Radiographs
  - PA, lateral, and oblique wrist:
    - Perilunate dislocation will show disruption of Gilula's lines with a loss of carpal height.
    - Lateral view may show dislocation of the capitate or lunate.

D. Classification

- As described by Mayfield et al (1980) and Herzberg et al (1993).

E. Management

1. Initial Management

- Reduction of any carpal dislocation
  - Usually requires complete muscular relaxation, axial traction, and recreation of initial injury mechanism followed by reduction.
  - Dorsal dislocation: Thumb should be placed volarly to prevent conversion to a volar lunate dislocation.
- Prompt surgical management
  - Nonoperative management is not advised: Persistent carpal instability, pain, weakness, and delayed surgical management result in worse outcomes.

2. Methods of Surgical Management

- Approaches:
  - Dorsal midline with or without volar component:
    - Arthroscopy can be useful; further diagnose ligamentous injuries, assess chondral injuries, and assist with reduction.
  - Specific injury patterns and their management
    - Greater arch injuries: Reduction of fracture typically required; usually scaphoid; 95% of fractures will be in middle third; amenable to cannulated screw, but may require bone grafting if comminuted.
    - Ligamentous injuries: Scapholunate interosseous ligament (SLIL)—suture anchor with Kirschner wire (K-wire); lunotriquetral interosseous ligament (LTIL)—suture anchor with K-wire.

3. Outcomes

- Studies on long-term outcomes for perilunate instability are limited to case series with varying methods of treatment.

○ In a study by Krief E et al (2015) on perilunate dislocations with minimum 18 years follow-up, 70% of patients developed radiographic arthritis.
  – Clinical and functional outcomes did not correlate with radiographic arthritis.
  – There was also a loss of ROM of wrist with an average arc of 90 degrees (35–140 degrees).

III. Triquetrum

A. Background

- Triquetral fractures are uncommon, but after scaphoid fractures, they are the second most common isolated carpal fractures.
  ○ Up to 15% of carpal fractures.
- Mechanism
  ○ Typically result from a fall onto an outstretched hand with wrist in dorsiflexion and ulnar in deviation.
    – Ligament avulsion fractures: Both intrinsic and extrinsic ligaments attach to triquetrum; thus many different ligaments are implicated. Volar avulsions are typically avulsions of the palmar ulnar triquetral or the lunotriquetral ligament.
    – Direct compression: Compression against ulnar styloid or hamate.

B. Presentation

- Focal tenderness on the dorsum of the triquetrum after a fall.

C. Evaluation

1. Radiographs

- PA, lateral, and oblique radiographs of the hand.
- 45 degrees pronated oblique view
  ○ Will view the triquetrum on profile
    – Can be especially helpful with dorsal fractures.
- Radial deviation
  ○ May be useful for volar avulsion fractures.

2. CT

- Has seen increased usage for fracture characterization and diagnosis confirmation.

D. Management

1. Nonoperative

- Dorsal chip fractures
  ○ Cast immobilization for 4 to 6 weeks at the most; rich vascular supply; low rate of complications.
- Volar avulsions
  ○ Mainstay of treatment involves management of potential carpal instability through cast immobilization and not the avulsion itself.

2. Operative

- Specific indications are sparse in the literature and clouded by other associated injuries.
- Determined based on the presence of associated injuries as well as degree of fracture displacement.
  - Typically reserved for triquetral body fractures:
    - Herbert compression screw.
    - K-wires.
- Some associated triangular fibrocartilage complex tears have been associated with dorsal triquetral fractures, and are potentially amenable to repair if patient notes persistent ulnar sided pain after bony healing has occurred.

IV. Trapezium

A. Background

- Third most common carpal fracture:
  - It forms 1 to 5% of all carpal fractures.
- Associated injuries may include other carpal fractures, carpometacarpal (CMC) dislocation, Bennett's fracture, and others.

B. Presentation

- Usually associated with point tenderness over the trapezium although case reports describe some patients with only minor base of thumb pain.
- Some patients have significant restriction of movement with swelling and ecchymosis.

C. Evaluation

1. Radiographs

- PA, lateral, and oblique radiographs of the hand.
- Robert's anteroposterior (AP) view:
  - Hand in full pronation; thus puts the trapezium on plane with the radiograph.
- Carpal tunnel view:
  - Can be useful for trapezial ridge fractures.

2. CT

- Useful if radiographs cannot confirm the diagnosis, or to further characterize the fracture fragments and articular surface involvement.

D. Classification

- Five main fracture patterns identified, each resulting from different mechanism:
  - Vertical intra-articular
    - Most common: Axial compression force from the thumb metacarpal.
  - Horizontal
    - Horizontal load against trapezium.

○ Dorsal radial tuberosity
  – Vertical shear between the radial styloid and the metacarpal.
○ Anterior medial ridge
  – Axial load of an avulsion of the transverse carpal ligament.
○ Comminuted
  – Relatively higher energy mechanism.

E. Management

- Nonoperative
  ○ Successful cast immobilization in case reports of most nondisplaced trapezium fractures.
- Operative
  ○ Many authors advocate open reduction and internal fixation if articular surface is involved, or displacement is greater than 2 mm; vertically displaced intra-articular fractures.
    – Most commonly described in literature.
    – Herbert screw or K-wires.

V. Capitate

A. Background

- Rare fractures
  ○ Approximately 1 to 2% of all carpal fractures.
- Likely, these fractures occur with other injuries due to the capitate's central location in the carpus.
  ○ Most common associated injury is a transscaphoid, transcapitate greater arch perilunate injury.
- Mechanism
  ○ Fall onto an extended wrist in ulnar deviation.
  ○ Can also occur through a direct axial load from the third metacarpal base.

B. Presentation

- The most common location for tenderness is at the dorsal, central wrist.

C. Evaluation

- Most have some element of a transverse fracture line.
  ○ General classifications:
    – Body fractures.
    – Avulsion tip.
    – Shear depression.
  ○ Fracture orientation specific classifications:
    – Transverse pole.
    – Transverse body.
    – Verticofrontal.
    – Parasagittal.

D. Management

- Management depends on the extent of the fracture, its location, and associated injuries:
  - Urgent reduction needed if associated with perilunate dislocation as described above.
- Literature is sparse regarding specific indications for operative fixation not including perilunate fracture/dislocations:
  - If nondisplaced, a fracture can be treated nonoperatively with cast immobilization.
  - Operative intervention usually consists of a headless compression screw or K-wires.

E. Complications

- Nonunion, osteonecrosis, and post-traumatic arthritis have all been reported.
  - Nonunion and osteonecrosis are traditionally attributed to the retrograde blood flow to the proximal pole, which can occur in a transverse body fracture.
    - Questionable rates of osteonecrosis with 30% rates shown in some case series, although more recent literature describes zero cases of osteonecrosis in a 23-patient cohort with limited 6 months follow-up.

VI. Hamate

A. Background

- Rare, accounting for 2% of all carpal fractures
  - High incidence of misdiagnosis
    - Bishop AT (1988) reported that in a series of 17 patients who initially sought medical attention for a later diagnosed hook fracture, only two cases were diagnosed by the initial evaluating physician.
- Hook of the hamate is a palmarly curved process that serves as the attachment point to the flexor carpi ulnaris, flexor digiti minimi, and opponens digiti minimi
  - It can be palpated approximately 2 cm distal along an imaginary line from the pisiform to the second metacarpal head.
- Mechanism
  - Hook fractures are increasingly being seen in club sport athletes
    - Likely repeated micro-trauma to the hypothenar eminence from the racket or club.
  - Body fractures can occur with punching injuries or with a dorsopalmar compression force at the wrist between heavy weights
    - Associated with dorsal carpal-metacarpal dislocations of the fourth and fifth metacarpals.

B. Presentation

- Vague hypothenar related pain without a specific inciting event.
- Tenderness on direct palpation over the hook or pain with resisted flexion of the ring and small fingers can help to confirm the diagnosis.
- Paresthesia or weakness in the ulnar distribution.

○ Hook is in close proximity to both the sensory and deep motor branches of the ulnar nerve.

C. Evaluation

1. Radiographs

- PA, lateral, and oblique radiographs of the hand
  ○ PA projection and lateral radiographs found to have false negative in 42.8 and 92.9%, respectively, of hook fractures.
- Supinated oblique (carpal tunnel view)
  ○ Can increase visualization.

2. CT

- Becoming increasingly more utilized.

D. Classification

- Hook of the hamate fractures
  ○ More common.
- Body fractures.

E. Management

- Nonoperative
  ○ Casting for nondisplaced fractures of body or hook.
- Operative
  ○ Excision of displaced hook.
  ○ Open reduction and internal fixation for displaced body fractures or those associated with dislocations:
    – Screw fixation for hamate fracture.
    – Consider K-wire pinning of CMC joints.

VII. Patient Case Reports

A. Patient 1

This is a 25-year-old right-hand-dominant male who presented for initial consultation secondary to a mechanical fall landing on his dominant hand. He landed on the dorsal side of his hand 2 days prior to evaluation in the hand clinic. He was found to have dislocations of his ring, small CMC articulations as well as hamate and capitate fractures. Prior to arrival he presented with a CT scan which demonstrated dorsally displaced, coronally oriented, intra-articular fracture through the dorsal capitate and central hamate. These were closed injuries without neurovascular compromise (▶ Fig. 7.1 and ▶ Fig. 7.2). He was subsequently taken to the operating room.

In the operating room, an incision was made over the fourth metacarpal base. Once the fracture site was exposed and reduced provisionally, a 1.5 mm plate was cut in half with half to fit to capitate and half to fit to hamate. Nonlocking screws were placed to provide compression. After reduction of the capitate and hamate, attention was paid to

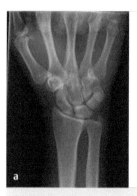
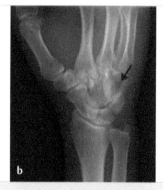
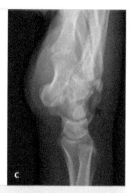

Fig. 7.1 (a–c) Posteroanterior (PA), oblique, and lateral images of right wrist demonstrating dislocations of the ring, small carpometacarpal articulations as well as hamate and capitate fractures.

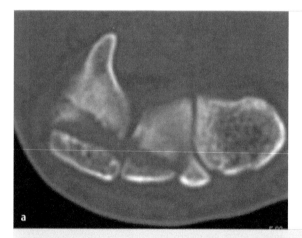
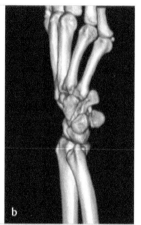

Fig. 7.2 (a) Axial CT images demonstrating the dorsally displaced capitate and hamate fractures. (b) Three-dimensional reconstructed image of the carpus demonstrating fracture-dislocation of ring and small fingers.

the CMC dislocation. Two transverse 0.045 K-wires connected the long, ring, and small fingers. Fluoroscopic images demonstrated adequate reduction and relocation. He was made non-weight-bearing and placed in an ulnar gutter splint. He was transitioned to a short arm cast at 2 weeks (▶ Fig. 7.3) with removal of the cast and pins at 6 weeks (▶ Fig. 7.4). He had no complications.

B. Patient 2

This is right-hand-dominant 44-year-old male who sustained an injury to his right hand approximately 5 to 6 weeks prior to evaluation after a mechanical fall. He was found to have a small finger CMC fracture-dislocation, as well as a hamate body

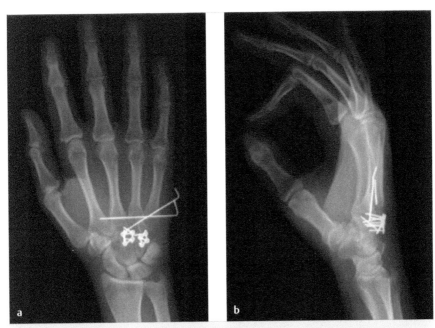

Fig. 7.3 (a, b) Posteroanterior (PA) and lateral images demonstrating fixation at 2 weeks postoperatively.

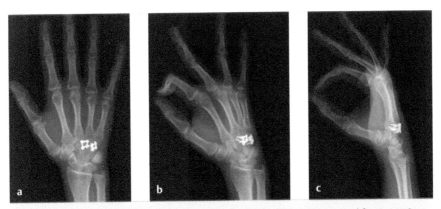

Fig. 7.4 (a–c) Posteroanterior (PA), oblique, and lateral images showing retained fixation at 3 months postoperatively with interval K-wire removal.

fracture (▶ Fig. 7.5). He was evaluated at our emergency department at the time of injury, but did not have insurance, thus delaying operative intervention. At the time of operation, a longitudinal incision was made over the base of the fourth and fifth CMC joints and hamate. The capsule over the fifth CMC joint was opened and the fracture-dislocation identified. The fifth CMC joint was reduced and pinned in place between the fifth, fourth, and third metacarpals using two 0.045 K-wires. The fracture of the

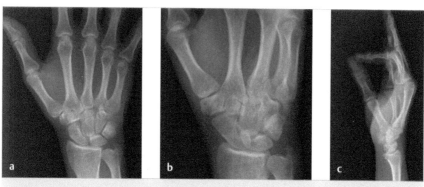

Fig. 7.5 (a–c) Posteroanterior (PA), oblique, and lateral images of right wrist demonstrating small finger dislocation with associated hamate body fracture.

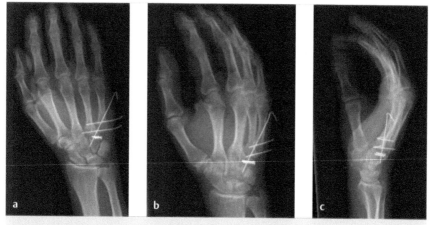

Fig. 7.6 (a–c) Posteroanterior (PA), oblique, and lateral images of right wrist demonstrating fixation at 2 weeks postoperatively.

hamate was opened and cleared of fracture hematoma, and then was open reduced, and two 2.0 mm screws were drilled and placed across the fracture. He was made non-weight-bearing and placed in an ulnar gutter splint. He was transitioned to a short arm cast at 2 weeks (▶ Fig. 7.6) with removal of the cast and pins at 6 weeks (▶ Fig. 7.7). He had no complications.

C. Patient 3

This is a right-hand-dominant 27-year-old male who sustained an injury to his left wrist when he was running and tripped and fell, and landed onto an outstretched hand. He was evaluated in the emergency department and then presented to the hand clinic 1 week later.

At our office, he arrived with a CT scan showing a trapezium fracture with intra-articular extension with significant displacement as well as a displaced hook of hamate

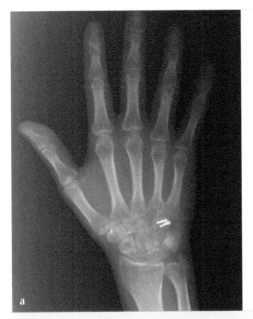
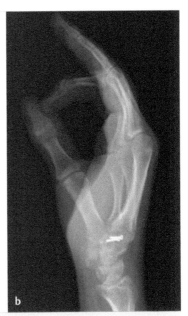

Fig. 7.7 (a, b) Posteroanterior (PA) and lateral images of right wrist demonstrating retained fixation at 3 months postoperatively with interval K-wire removal.

fracture (▶ Fig. 7.8). Given these characteristics, he elected for trapezium fixation and hook of the hamate excision due to the high risk of nonunion and chance of ulnar digit flexor tendon difficulty. A Wagner approach was made at the left thenar eminence, and after further exposure, the intra-articular nature of the fracture was visualized. The fracture was reduced and a micro screw was placed transversely across the fracture site after pre-drilling, providing compression across the fracture. There was a fracture on the volar and ulnar aspect of the trapezium at the ridge where the flexor carpi radialis (FCR) comes across; however, these were comminuted and small pieces, and these were excised to prevent tendon injury. The CMC joint was stable to shuck. Attention was then paid to the hook of the hamate where a longitudinal incision beginning at Kaplan cardinal line in line with the ulnar aspect of the ring finger ray and traveling proximally with the Bruner incision across the wrist was made.

The hook was excised leaving a smooth base. After appropriate closure, the patient was placed into a thumb spica splint. He transitioned to a thumb spica cast at 2 weeks (▶ Fig. 7.9) and remained immobilized until his 6-week visit (▶ Fig. 7.10). He had no complications.

D. Patient 4

This is a right-hand-dominant 18-year-old male who presented to the emergency department with right hand pain after he punched a wall. He later presented to orthopedic clinic 4 days later with a closed right transverse fourth metacarpal shaft fracture, fifth CMC dislocation, and hamate body fracture (▶ Fig. 7.11). He was neurovascularly intact. He was taken to the operating room the following week. At that time, open

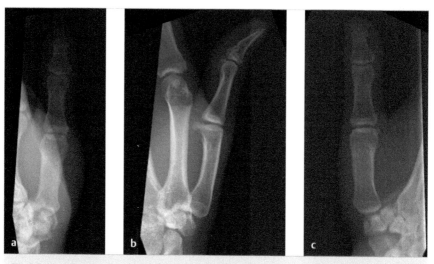

Fig. 7.8 (a–c) Posteroanterior (PA), lateral, and carpometacarpal (CMC) view of left hand demonstrating a displaced, transverse trapezium fracture.

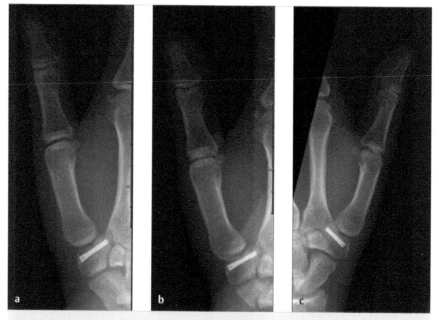

Fig. 7.9 (a–c) Robert's views of left hand demonstrating a headless compression screw through the trapezium fracture.

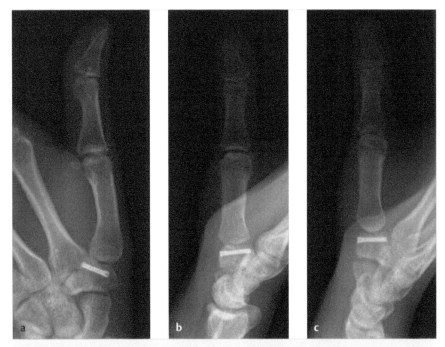

Fig. 7.10 (a–c) Lateral thumb and Robert's views of left hand demonstrating a headless compression screw through the trapezium fracture at 3 months postoperatively.

reduction internal fixation of the fourth metacarpal shaft and hamate was performed. The transverse orientation of the metacarpal shaft fracture was amenable to intramedullary pin that was buried. Percutaneous reduction of the fifth CMC dislocation was achieved with two 0.045 K-wires. He was immobilized in an ulnar gutter splint and made non-weight-bearing. He was transitioned to a short arm cast at 2 weeks (▶ Fig. 7.12) with removal of the cast and pins at 6 weeks (▶ Fig. 7.13). He had no complications.

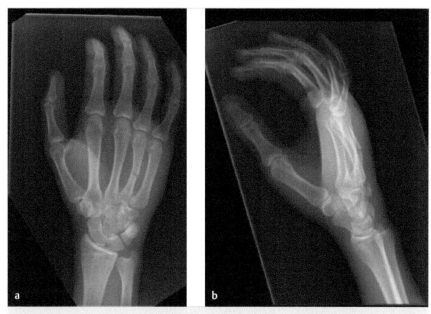

Fig. 7.11 (a, b) Posteroanterior (PA) and lateral views of hand demonstrating closed right transverse fourth metacarpal shaft fracture, fifth carpometacarpal (CMC) dislocation, and dorsal hamate body fracture.

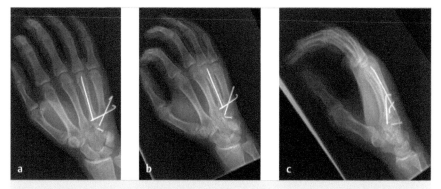

Fig. 7.12 (a–c) Posteroanterior (PA), oblique, and lateral views of hand demonstrating interval fixation at 2 weeks postoperatively.

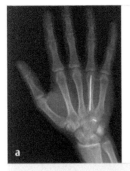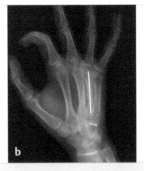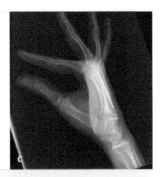

Fig. 7.13 (a–c) Posteroanterior (PA), oblique, and lateral views of hand demonstrating retained internal fixation at 3 months postoperatively with interval removal of K-wires.

Suggested Readings

Abboud JA, Beredjiklian PK, Bozentka DJ. Nonunion of a triquetral body fracture. A case report. J Bone Joint Surg Am. 2003; 85(12):2441–2444

Alnaeem H, Aldekhayel S, Kanevsky J, Neel OF. A systematic review and meta-analysis examining the differences between nonsurgical management and percutaneous fixation of minimally and nondisplaced scaphoid fractures. J Hand Surg Am. 2016; 41(12):1135–1144.e1

Amadio PC, Berquist TH, Smith DK, Ilstrup DM, Cooney WP, III, Linscheid RL. Scaphoid malunion. J Hand Surg Am. 1989; 14(4):679–687

Apergis E, Darmanis S, Kastanis G, Papanikolaou A. Does the term scaphocapitate syndrome need to be revised? A report of 6 cases. J Hand Surg [Br]. 2001; 26(5):441–445

Apostolides JG, Lifchez SD, Christy MR. Complex and rare fracture patterns in perilunate dislocations. Hand (N Y). 2011; 6(3):287–294

Arora S, Goyal A, Mittal S, Singh A, Sural S, Dhal A. Combined intraarticular fracture of the body and the hook of hamate: an unusual injury pattern. J Hand Microsurg. 2013; 5(2):92–95

Bachoura A, Wroblewski A, Jacoby SM, Osterman AL, Culp RW. Hook of hamate fractures in competitive baseball players. Hand (N Y). 2013; 8(3):302–307

Becce F, Theumann N, Bollmann C, et al. Dorsal fractures of the triquetrum: MRI findings with an emphasis on dorsal carpal ligament injuries. AJR Am J Roentgenol. 2013; 200(3):608–617

Berger RA. The anatomy of the scaphoid. Hand Clin. 2001; 17(4):525–532

Bishop AT, Beckenbaugh RD. Fracture of the hamate hook. J Hand Surg Am. 1988; 13(1):135–139

Bonnin JG, Greening WP. Fractures of the triquetrum. Br J Surg. 1944; 31:278–283

Borgeskov S, Christiansen B, Kjaer A, Balslev I. Fractures of the carpal bones. Acta Orthop Scand. 1966; 37(3):276–287

Budoff JE. Treatment of acute lunate and perilunate dislocations. J Hand Surg Am. 2008; 33(8):1424–1432

Buijze GA, Goslings JC, Rhemrev SJ, et al. CAST Trial Collaboration. Cast immobilization with and without immobilization of the thumb for nondisplaced and minimally displaced scaphoid waist fractures: a multicenter, randomized, controlled trial. J Hand Surg Am. 2014; 39(4):621–627

Burleson A, Shin S. Return to play after hook of hamate excision in baseball players. Orthop J Sports Med. 2018; 6(10):2325967118803090

Carroll RE, Lakin JF. Fracture of the hook of the hamate: acute treatment. J Trauma. 1993; 34(6):803–805

Chen NC, Jupiter JB, Jebson PJ. Sports-related wrist injuries in adults. Sports Health. 2009; 1(6):469–477

Chow JC, Weiss MA, Gu Y. Anatomic variations of the hook of hamate and the relationship to carpal tunnel syndrome. J Hand Surg Am. 2005; 30(6):1242–1247

Clementson M, Jørgsholm P, Besjakov J, Thomsen N, Björkman A. Conservative treatment versus arthroscopic-assisted screw fixation of scaphoid waist fractures—a randomized trial with minimum 4-year follow-up. J Hand Surg Am. 2015; 40(7):1341–1348

Clementson M, Thomsen N, Besjakov J, Jørgsholm P, Björkman A. Long-term outcomes after distal scaphoid fractures: a 10-year follow-up. J Hand Surg Am. 2017; 42(11):927.e1–927.e7

Cooney WP, Bussey R, Dobyns JH, Linscheid RL. Difficult wrist fractures: perilunate fracture-dislocations of the wrist. Clin Orthop Relat Res. 1987(214):136–147

Cordrey LJ, Ferrer-Torells M. Management of fractures of the greater multangular. Report of five cases. J Bone Joint Surg Am. 1960; 42-A:1111–1118

David TS, Zemel NP, Mathews PV. Symptomatic, partial union of the hook of the hamate fracture in athletes. Am J Sports Med. 2003; 31(1):106–111

Devers BN, Douglas KC, Naik RD, Lee DH, Watson JT, Weikert DR. Outcomes of hook of hamate fracture excision in high-level amateur athletes. J Hand Surg Am. 2013; 38(1):72–76

Dodds SD, Panjabi MM, Slade JF, III. Screw fixation of scaphoid fractures: a biomechanical assessment of screw length and screw augmentation. J Hand Surg Am. 2006; 31(3):405–413

Duckworth AD, Buijze GA, Moran M, et al. Predictors of fracture following suspected injury to the scaphoid. J Bone Joint Surg Br. 2012; 94(7):961–968

Durbin FC. Non-union of the triquetrum; report of a case. J Bone Joint Surg Br. 1950; 32-B(3):388

Failla JM. Hook of hamate vascularity: vulnerability to osteonecrosis and nonunion. J Hand Surg Am. 1993; 18(6):1075–1079

Foster RJ, Hastings H, II. Treatment of Bennett, Rolando, and vertical intraarticular trapezial fractures. Clin Orthop Relat Res. 1987(214):121–129

Fowler JR, Hughes TB. Scaphoid fractures. Clin Sports Med. 2015; 34(1):37–50

Garala K, Taub NA, Dias JJ. The epidemiology of fractures of the scaphoid: impact of age, gender, deprivation and seasonality. Bone Joint J. 2016; 98-B(5):654–659

Garcia-Elias M. Dorsal fractures of the triquetrum-avulsion or compression fractures? J Hand Surg Am. 1987; 12(2):266–268

Geissler WB. Arthroscopic management of scaphoid fractures in athletes. Hand Clin. 2009; 25(3):359–369

Gelberman RH, Vance RM, Zakaib GS. Fractures at the base of the thumb: treatment with oblique traction. J Bone Joint Surg Am. 1979; 61(2):260–262

Geurts G, van Riet R, Meermans G, Verstreken F. Incidence of scaphotrapezial arthritis following volar percutaneous fixation of nondisplaced scaphoid waist fractures using a transtrapezial approach. J Hand Surg Am. 2011; 36(11):1753–1758

Goodwin J, Castañeda P, Drace P, Edwards S. A biomechanical comparison of screw and plate fixations for scaphoid fractures. J Wrist Surg. 2018; 7(1):77–80

Grewal R, Suh N, MacDermid JC. Is casting for non-displaced simple scaphoid waist fracture effective? A CT based assessment of union. Open Orthop J. 2016b; 10:431–438

Guha AR, Marynissen H. Stress fracture of the hook of the hamate. Br J Sports Med. 2002; 36(3):224–225

Herzberg G, Comtet JJ, Linscheid RL, Amadio PC, Cooney WP, Stalder J. Perilunate dislocations and fracture-dislocations: a multicenter study. J Hand Surg Am. 1993; 18(5):768–779

Hey HW, Chong AK, Murphy D. Prevalence of carpal fracture in Singapore. J Hand Surg Am. 2011; 36(2):278–283

Inston N, Pimpalnerkar AL, Arafa MA. Isolated fracture of the trapezium: an easily missed injury. Injury. 1997; 28(7):485–488

Ivy AD, Stern PJ. Hamate hook and pisiform fractures. Oper Tech Sports Med. 2016; 24:94–99

Jethanandani RG, Rancy SK, Corpus KT, Yao J, Wolfe SW. Management of isolated capitate nonunion: a case series and literature review. J Wrist Surg. 2018; 7(5):419–423

Kang KB, Kim HJ, Park JH, Shin YS. Comparison of dorsal and volar percutaneous approaches in acute scaphoid fractures: a meta-analysis. PLoS One. 2016; 11(9):e0162779

Knoll VD, Allan C, Trumble TE. Trans-scaphoid perilunate fracture dislocations: results of screw fixation of the scaphoid and lunotriquetral repair with a dorsal approach. J Hand Surg Am. 2005; 30(6):1145–1152

Krief E, Appy-Fedida B, Rotari V, David E, Mertl P, Maes-Clavier C. Results of perilunate dislocations and perilunate fracture dislocations with a minimum 15-year follow-up. J Hand Surg Am. 2015; 40(11):2191–2197

Lee SJ, Rathod CM, Park KW, Hwang JH. Persistent ulnar-sided wrist pain after treatment of triquetral dorsal chip fracture: six cases related to triangular fibrocartilage complex injury. Arch Orthop Trauma Surg. 2012; 132(5):671–676

Linscheid RL, Dobyns JH, Beabout JW, Bryan RS. Traumatic instability of the wrist: diagnosis, classification, and pathomechanics. J Bone Joint Surg Am. 1972; 54(8):1612–1632

Mallee WH, Henny EP, van Dijk CN, Kamminga SP, van Enst WA, Kloen P. Clinical diagnostic evaluation for scaphoid fractures: a systematic review and meta-analysis. J Hand Surg Am. 2014; 39(9):1683–1691.e2

Mallee WH, Wang J, Poolman RW, et al. Computed tomography versus magnetic resonance imaging versus bone scintigraphy for clinically suspected scaphoid fractures in patients with negative plain radiographs. Cochrane Database Syst Rev. 2015; 6(6):CD010023

Mayfield JK, Johnson RP, Kilcoyne RK. Carpal dislocations: pathomechanics and progressive perilunar instability. J Hand Surg Am. 1980; 5(3):226–241

McCallister WV, Knight J, Kaliappan R, Trumble TE. Central placement of the screw in simulated fractures of the scaphoid waist: a biomechanical study. J Bone Joint Surg Am. 2003; 85(1):72–77

McGuigan FX, Culp RW. Surgical treatment of intra-articular fractures of the trapezium. J Hand Surg Am. 2002; 27(4):697–703

McQueen MM, Gelbke MK, Wakefield A, Will EM, Gaebler C. Percutaneous screw fixation versus conservative treatment for fractures of the waist of the scaphoid: a prospective randomised study. J Bone Joint Surg Br. 2008; 90(1):66–71

Monahan PR, Galasko CS. The scapho-capitate fracture syndrome: a mechanism of injury. J Bone Joint Surg Br. 1972; 54(1):122–124

Monahan PR, Galasko CS. The scapho-capitate fracture syndrome: a mechanism of injury. J Bone Joint Surg Br 1972;54(1):122–124

Nguyen Q, Chaudhry S, Sloan R, Bhoora I, Willard C. The clinical scaphoid fracture: early computed tomography as a practical approach. Ann R Coll Surg Engl. 2008; 90(6):488–491

Noordman BJ, Hartholt KA, Halm JA. Simultaneous, bilateral fracture of the triquetral bone. BMJ Case Rep. 2015; 2015:bcr2015212133

Parvizi J, Wayman J, Kelly P, Moran CG. Combining the clinical signs improves diagnosis of scaphoid fractures: a prospective study with follow-up. J Hand Surg [Br]. 1998; 23(3):324–327

Pointu J, Schwenck JP, Destree G, Séjourné P. [Fractures of the trapezium. Mechanisms. Anatomo-pathology and therapeutic indications]. Rev Chir Orthop Repar Appar Mot. 1988; 74(5):454–465

Putnam MDM, Meyer NJ. Carpal Fractures Excluding the Scaphoid. Rosemont, IL: American Society for Surgery of the Hand; 2003

Ramoutar DN, Katevu C, Titchener AG, Patel A. Trapezium fracture—a common technique to fix a rare injury: a case report. Cases J. 2009; 2:8304

Rand JA, Linscheid RL, Dobyns JH. Capitate fractures: a long-term follow-up. Clin Orthop Relat Res. 1982(165):209–216

Rocchi L, Fanfani F, Pagliei A, Catalano F. [Treatment of scaphoid waist fractures by shape memory staples. Retrospective evaluation on 60 cases]. Chir Main. 2005; 24(3–4):153–160

Rua T, Parkin D, Goh V, McCrone P, Gidwani S. The economic evidence for advanced imaging in the diagnosis of suspected scaphoid fractures: systematic review of evidence. J Hand Surg Eur Vol. 2018; 43(6):642–651

Russe O. Fracture of the carpal navicular: diagnosis, non-operative treatment, and operative treatment. J Bone Joint Surg Am 1960;42-A:759–768

Sabat D, Arora S, Dhal A. Isolated capitate fracture with dorsal dislocation of proximal pole: a case report. Hand (N Y). 2011; 6(3):333–336

Scheufler O, Kamusella P, Tadda L, Radmer S, Russo SG, Andresen R. High incidence of hamate hook fractures in underwater rugby players: diagnostic and therapeutic implications. Hand Surg. 2013; 18(3):357–363

Scheufler O, Radmer S, Andresen R. Dorsal percutaneous cannulated mini-screw fixation for fractures of the hamate hook. Hand Surg. 2012; 17(2):287–293

Shammas RL, Mela N, Wallace S, Tong BC, Huber J, Mithani SK. Conjoint analysis of treatment preferences for non-displaced scaphoid fractures. J Hand Surg Am. 2018; 43(7):678.e1–678.e9

Sin CH, Leung YF, Ip SP, Wai YL, Ip WY. Non-union of the triquetrum with pseudoarthrosis: a case report. J Orthop Surg (Hong Kong). 2012; 20(1):105–107

Stark HH, Chao EK, Zemel NP, Rickard TA, Ashworth CR. Fracture of the hook of the hamate. J Bone Joint Surg Am. 1989; 71(8):1202–1207

Suh N, Ek ET, Wolfe SW. Carpal fractures. J Hand Surg Am. 2014; 39(4):785–791, quiz 791

Suzuki T, Nakatsuchi Y, Tateiwa Y, Tsukada A, Yotsumoto N. Osteochondral fracture of the triquetrum: a case report. J Hand Surg Am. 2002; 27(1):98–100

Tait MA, Bracey JW, Gaston RG. Acute scaphoid fractures: a critical analysis review. JBJS Rev. 2016; 4(9):01874474-201609000-00004

Temple CL, Ross DC, Bennett JD, Garvin GJ, King GJ, Faber KJ. Comparison of sagittal computed tomography and plain film radiography in a scaphoid fracture model. J Hand Surg Am. 2005; 30(3):534–542

Ten Berg PW, Drijkoningen T, Strackee SD, Buijze GA. Classifications of acute scaphoid fractures: a systematic literature review. J Wrist Surg. 2016; 5(2):152–159

Trumble TE, Clarke T, Kreder HJ. Non-union of the scaphoid: treatment with cannulated screws compared with treatment with Herbert screws. J Bone Joint Surg Am. 1996; 78(12):1829–1837

Van Schil P, De Smet C. Simultaneous fracture of carpal scaphoid and trapezium. J Hand Surg [Br]. 1986; 11(1):112–114

Vander Grend R, Dell PC, Glowczewskie F, Leslie B, Ruby LK. Intraosseous blood supply of the capitate and its correlation with aseptic necrosis. J Hand Surg Am. 1984; 9(5):677–683

Verstreken F, Meermans G. Transtrapezial approach for fixation of acute scaphoid fractures: rationale, surgical techniques and results: AAOS exhibit selection. J Bone Joint Surg Am. 2015; 97(10):850–858

Walker JL, Greene TL, Lunseth PA. Fractures of the body of the trapezium. J Orthop Trauma. 1988; 2(1):22–28

Walsh JJ, IV, Bishop AT. Diagnosis and management of hamate hook fractures. Hand Clin. 2000; 16(3):397–403, viii

Weil WM, Slade JF, III, Trumble TE. Open and arthroscopic treatment of perilunate injuries. Clin Orthop Relat Res. 2006; 445(445):120–132

Weum S, Millerjord S, de Weerd L. The distribution of hand fractures at the university hospital of north Norway. J Plast Surg Hand Surg. 2016; 50(3):146–150

Yin ZG, Zhang JB, Kan SL, Wang XG. Diagnostic accuracy of imaging modalities for suspected scaphoid fractures: meta-analysis combined with latent class analysis. J Bone Joint Surg Br. 2012; 94(8):1077–1085

8 Fractures and Dislocations of the Distal Radius and Ulna

Eric Schafer, Benjamin K. Gundlach, and Jeffrey N. Lawton

Abstract

Fractures of the distal forearm are among the most common injuries treated by orthopaedic surgeons and hand surgeons. This chapter begins with distal radius fractures, first reviewing the epidemiology, classification, and evaluation. The operative indications and subsequent techniques are then discussed, focusing on important points of each treatment. Although open reduction and internal fixation is the most common operative treatment, there are many other modalities to be considered as well. Also included is a section on operative considerations of certain fracture patterns such as volar ulnar corner injuries and how they differ in management. Finally, the complications associated with distal radius fractures are reviewed.

Fractures of the distal ulna are discussed next. Although often seen in combination with distal radius fractures, ulnar fractures can occur in isolation. Again evaluation, classification, and management are reviewed, including a discussion of the controversy involving when to fix ulnar styloid fractures associated with a distal radius injury.

Lastly, Galleazzi fractures, or fractures of the distal radius with disruption of the distal radioulnar joint (DRUJ), are reviewed. The biomechanics of the DRUJ as well as appropriate imaging to help detect injury are discussed. In adults, Galleazzi fractures are invariably treated with surgery.

Keywords: Distal radius, distal ulna, ulnar styloid, fracture, galleazzi, distal radioulnar joint (DRUJ)

I. Distal Radius Fractures

A. Epidemiology

- Distal radius fractures are one of the most common fractures encountered by hand/upper extremity surgeons.
- In 2000, there were 1.7 million osteoporotic fractures of the forearm, followed by 1.6 million hip fractures.[1]
  - Occur in a 4:1 female to male ratio.[1]
- They carry a significant cost of treatment burden. In 2007, Medicare paid $170 million for distal radius fractures.[2]
- As with many other fractures, they occur in a bimodal age distribution with higher energy injuries occurring in younger patients and lower energy osteoporotic fractures occurring in the elderly.
- Distal radius fractures are important to recognize as they are predictors of subsequent osteoporotic fractures.[3]
  - The relative risk of a hip fracture is 1.54 in women and 2.27 in men with osteoporotic distal radius fractures.[4]

B. Evaluation

- As with all fractures, a thorough history and neurovascular/skin examination is paramount.
- Median nerve dysfunction is the most common nerve injury as a consequence of its proximity to the distal radius.[5]
  - The median nerve lies closer to the radius as it travels more distally and is estimated to be 3 mm or so from the bone at the level of the wrist.[6]
  - Incidence of acute carpal tunnel syndrome requiring decompression is estimated to be 3 to 9%.[5,7]
  - All patients should be asked about any history of carpal tunnel syndrome and any new/acute symptoms accompanying the injury.
- Imaging evaluation includes initial posteroanterior, lateral, and supplemental oblique X-rays.
  - Postreduction X-rays may include a modified lateral projection with the beam angled 10 degrees proximally to evaluate the reduction of the articular surface.[8]
  - Medoff published average radiographic parameters of the distal radius from a sample size of 40, including radial inclination (23.6 degrees), radial height (11.6 degrees), and volar tilt (11.2 degrees).[8] The normal radiographic parameters of the distal radius are shown in ▶ Fig. 8.1 (normal wrist X-ray with overlying parameters).
  - Forearm X-rays should also be included to evaluate the elbow as well.
  - It is important to inspect the distal radioulnar joint (DRUJ) to assess for concomitant injury.
- Lafontaine described criteria associated with unstable distal radius fractures which are therefore at risk of secondary displacement after reduction (▶ Table 8.1).[9]

C. Classification

- Historically there have been many published classification systems of distal radius fractures as listed in ▶ Table 8.2.[10] Details of each of these systems are beyond the scope of this chapter.
- For research purposes, the AO/Universal classification is most widely used today.
- Clinically, a descriptive classification of the fracture is often sufficient.

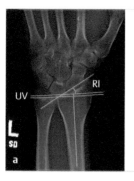 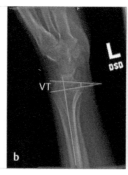

Fig. 8.1 Normal anteroposterior (AP) (a) and lateral (b) wrist X-ray with overlying parameters. RI, radial inclination; UV, ulnar variance; VT, volar tilt.

Table 8.1 LaFontaine criteria

Degree of dorsal displacement

Associated ulnar styloid fracture

Age >60 years

Dorsal comminution

Intra-articular involvement

Table 8.2 Classifications of distal radius fractures

Gartland and Werley	Lidstrom	Older and Colleagues
Thomas	Malone	Jenkins
McMurtry and Jupiter	Universal/AO	Mayo Clinic
Fernandez		

D. Treatment

1. Nonoperative Treatment

- Nondisplaced fractures are likely inherently stable and can be treated with removable bracing for protection.
- Closed reduction and splinting is indicated as the initial management for all displaced distal radius fractures presenting to the emergency room.
- Although controversial, evidence suggests that lower demand and/or elderly patients with mild residual deformity after closed reduction may still do well with nonoperative management in a cast.
  - The American Academy of Orthopaedic Surgeons (AAOS) guidelines are unable to recommend for or against operative treatment in patients older than 55.[11]
  - Chung et al found elderly patients tend to do well with either open reduction internal fixation (ORIF) or casting; however, ORIF was estimated to be seven times more expensive.[12]
- Casting techniques: The Cotton-Loder position of wrist flexion and ulnar deviation should be avoided as this has been shown to increase carpal tunnel pressure.
  - Gelberman et al showed increasing carpal tunnel pressure to 47 mmHg at 40 degrees of wrist flexion.[13]
- The AAOS guidelines recommend weekly radiographic follow-up for 3 weeks after injury to evaluate for fracture displacement.[11]

2. Closed Reduction and Percutaneous Pinning

- In young patients with extra-articular fractures, pinning alone is an option.
- Trumble et al demonstrated good results with pinning in fractures with comminution of only one cortex in young patients. Supplementary external fixation was required if comminution extended to two or more cortices.[14]
- In older patients with extra-articular and/or minimally displaced intra-articular fractures, pinning is also an option; however, it requires supplemental external or internal fixation.[14]

○ External fixation or internal bridging plate depends on the ligamentaxis to hold reduction.[15]

3. External Fixation

- Agee helped to popularize the idea of using an external fixator to achieve fracture reduction via multiplanar ligamentotaxis.[15]
- External fixation is often useful in situations with significant soft tissue compromise, polytrauma, highly comminuted articular fractures, etc.

4. Bridge Plating

- Hanel et al popularized bridge plating to act as an internal fixator (vs. external) for distal radius fractures.[16]
- Indications include high energy fractures with extension into the radial metaphysis and polytrauma patients requiring early use of the upper extremities.
- Although the original technique involved using a 3.5-mm plate on the floor of the 4th dorsal compartment to the 3rd metacarpal,[17] Hanel et al published a modification using either a Synthes 2.4 mm distal radius bridge plate or mandibular reconstruction plate through the 2nd dorsal compartment to the 2nd metacarpal (▶ Fig. 8.2).[16]
- The bridge plate functions as an internal fixator, reducing the fracture through ligamentotaxis.
- Advantages include reducing the need for nursing care of pin site tracts on external fixators, relatively short operative time, and a stable wrist to allow early use of the upper extremity.
  ○ Immediate weight bearing through the forearm and elbow is permissible with a platform walker followed by transition to hand grip crutches at 1 month or so.

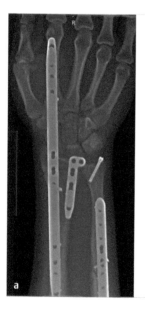
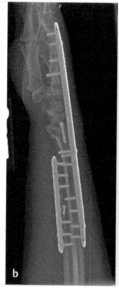

Fig. 8.2 (a, b) Plating of a distal radius fracture using a Synthes bridge plate. The patient presented with multiple injuries as well as an open fracture. Note the fragment-specific fixation of the dorsal ulnar corner of the distal radius as this was not supported by the bridge plate.

- The plate is removed after fracture consolidation, an average of 112 days in Hanel's series.[16]

5. Open Reduction and Internal Fixation: Volar Plating

- In the 1990s, Orbay introduced locked volar plating as an alternative to the more common dorsal plating at the time.[18] This was quickly adopted given the high rate of extensor tendon irritation/ruptures seen with dorsal plating.
- Volar plating has demonstrated improved functional results in the early postoperative period with few complications compared to other treatment methods.[19]
- Indications including unstable distal radius fractures, open fractures, and fractures failing nonoperative management.
  - The AAOS guidelines recommend operative fixation of fractures with postreduction radial shortening >3 mm, dorsal tilt >10 degrees, or intra-articular displacement/step-off >2 mm. However, the guidelines do not recommend for or against any specific type of operative treatment.[11]
- Approach to the distal radius (**Video 8.1**)
  - The fracture is most commonly accessed via the modified Henry approach to the distal radius, utilizing the interval between the median nerve/carpal tunnel contents and the radial artery—through the floor of the flexor carpi radialis sheath
  - This incision may be extended to further open the carpal tunnel should decompression be required.
  - The radial artery and the superficial branch of the medial nerve are at risk.
  - Although effort should be made to repair the horizontal limb of the pronator quadratus exposure in order to cover the plate, there were no differences in range of motion (ROM), grip strength, and postoperative complications in a series by Ahsan et al[20] which evaluated repair versus no repair of the pronator quadratus (PQ).
- Reduction techniques
  - In the operating room, the reduction maneuver of Agee can be utilized to recreate radial height, volar tilt, and intra-articular step-off via ligamentotaxis.[21]
  - Reduction maneuver involves traction, volar translation, and pronation.
  - Should the reduction be unstable, it can be pinned with K-wires aimed proximally through the radial styloid.
  - Additionally, weighted traction can be applied with finger traps off the edge of the table to provisionally hold the reduction while the plate is applied.
  - The plate itself can be used as a reduction tool to restore volar tilt as well. The plate is first attached distally such that the proximal portion sits off the radial diaphysis. Then bringing this proximal plate down to bone will tilt the articular surface volarly—"Lift-off" technique.
- Outcomes
  - Open reduction and internal fixation with volar fixed angle plating has been shown to provide a stable reduction and allow for earlier ROM.[22]
  - ORIF has also been shown to provide a quicker return to function.[19]

6. Fragment-Specific Fixation

- Fragment-specific fixation has shown to be a viable alternative to other forms of fixation in certain instances.[23]

- The benefits of this approach include versatile fixation that can be tailored to specific fracture patterns and strong fixation that allows for early postoperative ROM.[23,24]
  - Fragment-specific fixation has been shown to provide stronger fixation of volar ulnar corner fragments biomechanically.[25]
- Drawbacks include an initial learning curve that may increase operative times and hardware irritation.[23] In addition, missed fragments may result in an unstable fixation, highlighting the need for careful preoperative planning.
- Principles
  - There are five primary fracture elements that need to be addressed, namely, radial column, ulnar corner, volar rim, dorsal wall, and impacted articular fracture fragments.[26]
  - Commonly available pin and plate configurations include[26,27] volar pin plates, ulnar pin plates, radial pin/column plates, dorsal/volar buttress clip pins, and dorsal/volar radial hook plates.
  - Plates are placed in an orthogonal position to increase strength.[24,26]
  - The focus is on anatomic articular reduction.[24]
  - Metaphyseal defects are filled with bone graft in order to prevent loss of radial length.[24]
  - Small fragments may not need specific fixation if large fragments are fixed around them to hold in place.
  - Wrist ROM should be started early to prevent postoperative stiffness.[24,26]
- Approaches:
  - Volar approach:[26,27]
    - Although the extended flexor carpi radialis (FCR) approach allows access to the entire volar surface of the distal radius, more limited approaches may be used as well depending on the fracture pattern.
    - Limited-incision volar approach: Utilizes interval between radial artery and brachioradialis to gain access to the volar radial aspect of the distal radius.
    - Volar ulnar approach: Utilizes the interval between the flexor carpi ulnaris (FCU) and the flexor digitorum profundus (FDP) tendons to gain access to the volar ulnar corner of the distal radius.
  - Dorsal approach:
    - A standard 3rd compartment splitting approach may be utilized to view the entire dorsal surface of the radius if needed. Alternatively more limited approaches can be used.
    - Interval between the 3rd and 4th extensor compartments can be used to access the dorsal wall.
    - Interval between the 4th and 5th compartments can gain access to the dorsal ulnar corner as needed.
- Medoff suggests a stepwise operative approach that involves:[26]
  - Restoring radial column length.
  - Fixing the volar rim.
  - Reducing and fixing any dorsal or free articular components to the previously fixed volar rim, using bone graft as needed for defects.
  - Fixing with a radial column plate to maintain length.
- Contraindications[24]
  - Fracture fragment extension into the radial diaphysis is an absolute contraindication.

○ Relative contraindications include very poor quality bone and large metaphyseal defects.

7. Dorsal Plating

- Although historically associated with a greater rate of tendon irritation, dorsal plating may still be a viable option for certain fracture patterns.
  ○ Low profile dorsal plates have shown similar complication rates to volar plating at 1 year follow-up.[28]
  ○ Rozental et al showed it may be the low profile nature of the new dorsal locking plates that minimizes complications.[29]
- An unstable fracture pattern of the distal radius as a result of significant dorsal comminution is the main indication for dorsal plating.
  ○ Trease et al showed that dorsal plating constructs are twice as stiff with an approximately 50% higher load to failure than volar plating.[30]
- Main contraindications to dorsal plating include volar comminution resulting in volarly unstable fracture patterns and carpal tunnel syndrome (relative).
- Approach:
  ○ The dorsal distal radius is approached through the 3rd dorsal compartment, subperiosteally elevating for full exposure.

8. Vitamin C

- In 2007, Zollinger et al demonstrated that vitamin C can reduce the risk of complex regional pain syndrome (CRPS) in patients with distal radius fractures (2.4% vs. 10.1% in the placebo group).[31]
  ○ The recommended dose is 500 mg daily for 50 days.
- More recent evidence remains controversial with some studies finding no benefit[7,32] while others do support it.[33,34]
- Despite the controversy, the AAOS guidelines give a moderate strength recommendation for adjuvant use of vitamin C to prevent disproportionate pain.

E. Operative Considerations

1. Fractures of the Volar Ulnar Corner

- Fractures of the volar ulnar corner (involving the lunate facet) can lead to radiocarpal instability.[35]
- These fractures may not be captured with standard volar plating systems and may require fragment-specific plating in order to hold reduction (▶ Fig. 8.3).

2. Ligamentous Injuries

- Associated ligamentous injuries are quite common with distal radius fractures. In an arthroscopic series by Richards et al,[36] they found:
  ○ Torn triangular fibrocartilage complex (TFCC) in 35% of intra-articular and 53% of extra-articular distal radius fractures.
  ○ Scapholunate ligament instability in 21.5% of intra-articular and 6.7% of extra-articular fractures.

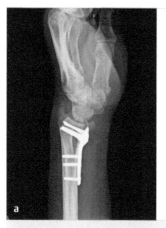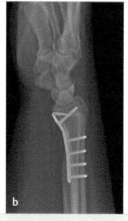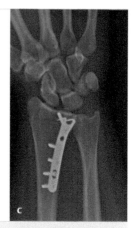

Fig. 8.3 **(a)** Loss of radiocarpal alignment after failure to support volar ulnar corner fragment. Note the volar subluxation of the carpus relative to the distal radius. **(b, c)** Appropriate fragment-specific fixation of volar ulnar corner in another patient.

- Lunotriquetral ligament instability in 6.7% of intra-articular and 13.3% of extra-articular fractures.

3. DRUJ Instability

- DRUJ instability may be present in approximately 11% of distal radius fractures.[37] It is important to recognize given the debilitating sequalae of an untreated injury.
- The diagnosis may be made with clinical correlation to the radiographs and/or on stress testing in the operating room.
- Treatment of unstable DRUJ injuries include pinning of the DRUJ or supination casting if pinning is not feasible.

F. Complications

- Arora et al reported an overall 27% complication rate with extensor and flexor tendon irritation accounting for the majority (57%).[38]

1. Extensor Tendon Rupture

- Extensor pollics longus (EPL) rupture is estimated to be approximately 5% in nondisplaced fractures.[39]
  - It is thought to be secondary to compartment syndrome-like phenomenon of the first dorsal compartment.
- Extensor tendon irritation can be caused by dorsal screw penetration.
  - Ozer et al compared four intraoperative fluoroscopic views and found that the standard lateral view was not sufficient to detect dorsal screw penetration.[40] Instead, the 45-degree supination view was the most sensitive for detecting penetration into the 2nd dorsal compartment. The tangential view was the most sensitive for

Table 8.3 Soong grade

Grade 0	Plate remains dorsal to the critical line extending from most volar aspect of the rim
Grade 1	Plate is volar to the critical line but remains proximal to the volar rim
Grade 2	Plate is volar to the critical line and is at or beyond the volar rim

the third dorsal compartment. Both the 45-degree pronation view and dorsal tangential view were most useful for the forth dorsal compartment.

2. Flexor Tendon Rupture

- In 2011, Soong et al published data showing three cases of flexor tendon ruptures (4%).[41] They developed the Soong grading system to evaluate plate prominence on the lateral wrist radiograph (▶ Table 8.3). Two of the three ruptures were Soong Grade 2 while the third was a Soong Grade 1.
  - Interestingly, all three cases of flexor tendon rupture occurred with the Acu-Loc plate (Accumed) which was designed to extend further distally and volarly on the radius. No cases of tendon rupture were seen with the DVR plating system (DePuy).
- Casaletto et al published a flexor pollicis longus (FPL) rupture rate of 1.9% at an average of 13.4 months.[42] They attributed the failure to technical factors—plate too distal, prominent screw heads, and the plate not being well seated.
- In 2017, Wolfe et al published risk factors for FPL rupture based on an anatomic model.[43] They showed that loss of volar tilt, wrist extension, and a higher Soong grade plate position resulted in greater contact between FPL and the plate.

3. Carpal Tunnel Syndrome

- The rate of acute carpal tunnel syndrome after ORIF of the distal radius is approximately 5.4%. Greater fracture translation in younger females has been shown to be a risk factor.[44]
- Ward et al published a 9% rate of paresthesias/numbness after volar plating with a 3% rate of carpal tunnel syndrome requiring release.[45]
- Immediate carpal tunnel release should be performed in a patient presenting with a distal radius fracture and symptoms of acute carpal tunnel syndrome persisting after reduction. In patients developing symptoms postoperatively, immediate release should be considered as well.

II. Distal Ulna Fractures

A. Epidemiology

- Distal ulna fractures, which we would consider any fracture that occurs within 4 cm of the distal aspect of the ulna, can occur with a variety of fracture patterns.
- Isolated distal ulna fractures are not as common as the distal radius fracture, and occur in isolation most commonly after direct blow to the distal ulna. Historically, these have been referred to as night-stick fractures.

- Distal ulna fractures, specifically ulnar styloid fractures, are commonly seen in combination with distal radius fractures, in fact occurring in up to 70% of distal radius fractures.[36] An isolated ulnar styloid fracture should raise suspicion for a DRUJ or TFCC injury.

B. Evaluation

- Standard radiographs of the wrist are sufficient to diagnose most distal ulna fractures; however, a computed tomography (CT) scan may be of use when evaluating for comminuted ulnar head fractures involving the chondral surface.
- Advanced imaging can also be of use when attempting to evaluate the soft tissue structures surrounding the ulnar side of the wrist. Through meta-analysis, Smith et al have shown that a magnetic resonance (MR) arthrogram of the wrist is the most sensitive and specific noninvasive test for evaluating TFCC pathology; 0.84 and 0.95 respectively. If MR arthrogram is unavailable, a standard magnetic resonance imaging (MRI) still has acceptable performance with a sensitivity and specificity of 0.75 and 0.81, respectively.[46]

C. Classification

- The AO classification is most commonly used clinically and for research purposes. If the distal ulna fractures are associated with a distal radius fracture, the AO Q Modification is used.

D. Treatment

1. Nonoperative Management

- Similar to distal radius fractures, minimally displaced fractures of the distal ulna especially in the elderly can be managed well with splint/cast treatment and close follow-up.
- Controversy exists in regard to when an ulnar styloid fracture with an associated distal radius fracture requires internal fixation. Given that the volar and dorsal distal radioulnar ligaments attach at the base of the ulnar styloid,[37] there is concern that displaced styloid fractures can create DRUJ instability. May et al. (2002) found that ulnar styloid base fractures, or a styloid fracture displaced greater than 2 mm, were associated with increased DRUJ instability.[47] Wijffels and Ring demonstrated that patients who were managed nonoperatively and developed an ulnar styloid nonunion were frequently asymptomatic, with preserved function and DRUJ stability when compared to patients with united fractures at 30 months.[48] Currently, the literature supports managing combined distal radius/ulnar styloid fractures with initial distal radius internal fixation—if DRUJ instability exists after radius fixation, then ulnar styloid fixation is recommended.[49]

2. Operative Management

- For isolated ulnar styloid fixation, we recommend either using a tension band (▶ Fig. 8.4), or headless compression screw construct (▶ Fig. 8.5). To date, there are no biomechanical studies proving superiority; however, a single pin + wire tension band is cheaper.

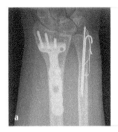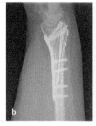

Fig. 8.4 (a, b) Ulnar styloid tension banding.

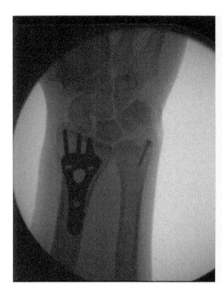

Fig. 8.5 Open reduction internal fixation (ORIF) of distal radius with ulnar styloid fixation.

- If a distal shaft and/or ulnar head fracture exists, it is recommended to use a distal ulna plate construct. There exists a variety of anatomy-specific plate options—some have an additional ulnar styloid hook and lay directly ulnar, while other plates lay on the anterior cortex.
- Regardless of your fixation, the approach to the distal ulna is most commonly gained through a direct medial/ulnar approach between the FCU and extensor carpi ulnaris (ECU). Take care to find and retract the dorsal sensory branch of the ulnar nerve, which branches off the medial aspect of the ulnar nerve and enters the subcutaneous tissue approximately 5 cm from the distal ulna.[50]

E. Operative Considerations

1. Measuring Ulnar Height

- When fixing distal ulna shaft/head fractures, if one is not careful there can be either an increase or decrease in ulnar height; the former can lead to ulnar abutment. To avoid this, we recommend having preoperative imaging of the contralateral wrist, with which to compare when deciding on ulnar height intraoperatively.

F. Complications

1. Neuropraxia

- As previously discussed, the dorsal sensory branch of the ulnar nerve is commonly encountered with distal ulna approaches, and postoperative neuropraxia is frequently experienced. In our experience this is usually transient.

2. Hardware Irritation

- Given the small amount of overlying soft issue, many plate constructs create hardware irritation necessitating removal.

III. Galeazzi Fractures

A. Definition

- The term Galeazzi fracture-dislocation refers to a fracture of the radius with disruption of DRUJ.
- Fractures of the distal radius and ulnar with DRUJ disruption is also a Galeazzi variant.
- This injury pattern was first described in the early 1800s although it gained its namesake after Galleazzi's series in 1934.[51,52]
- It is often referred to as a "fracture of necessity" in reference to the historically poor outcomes if not treated with surgery.[53,54,55]

B. Biomechanics of DRUJ

- Bony contact provides only an estimated 20% of DRUJ stability.[56]
  - The remaining stability is therefore provided by the soft tissue, mainly the TFCC. The TFCC is composed of: triangular fibrocartilage, ulnocarpal meniscus, dorsal radioulnar ligament, palmar radiolular ligament, and the subsheath of ECU.[57]
  - Of the multiple components of the TFCC, the dorsal and palmar radioulnar ligaments are thought to contribute most to DRUJ stability.[56]

C. Classification

- In 2001, Rettig and Raskin published data supporting classifying the radius fracture based on the distance from the wrist.[58]
  - Fractures <7.5 cm from the distal radius mid-articular surface were found to be associated with DRUJ instability in 55% of cases after ORIF of the radius.
  - Whereas fractures >7.5 cm away were only associated with a 6% rate of DRUJ instability.
- Ring et al also published data showing that the more distal the radius fractures occurred, the higher was the association with DRUJ instability.[59]
  - In a series including nine DRUJ injuries with radius fractures, they found five fractures occurred in the distal radius (56%), three in the middle radius (33%), and one in the proximal radius (11%).
- In 2011, Korompilias et al confirmed these associations as well.[60]

- Radius fractures were classified as type I (distal one-third), type II (middle one-third), and type III (proximal one-third).
- Fixation was required in 54% of type I radius fractures that had associated DRUJ instability while only 12% of type II and 11% of type III fractures required DRUJ stabilization.
- Bruckner et al suggested terming the DRUJ dislocation as either "simple" or "complex," depending upon whether soft tissue inhibited closed reduction.[61]

D. Mechanism of Injury

- Mechanism of injury is mainly thought to be secondary to hyperextension and pronation at the wrist.[55]
  - However, there is evidence that an axial blow which contributes >10 mm of radial shortening has shown to be associated with TFCC and interosseous membrane disruption.[62]

E. Imaging

- Forearm and wrist radiographs are required. Wrist radiographs include an anteroposterior (AP) and a lateral at minimum.
  - AP view is helpful to determine ulnar variance.
  - Greater than 5 mm of ulnar positive variance has been associated with DRUJ disruption in biomechanical studies.[63]
  - Lateral view can show DRUJ dislocation, which should be described as the radius' position in relation to the distal ulna as the ulna is the fixed element at the elbow.
  - The quality of the lateral radiograph at the wrist can be evaluated with the following criteria[64]:
    - Pisiform should be transected in half by palmar cortex of capitate.
    - Anterior cortex of distal pole of scaphoid should not extend beyond the pisiform.

F. Treatment

1. Nonoperative Treatment

- Galeazzi injuries have done notoriously poorly with nonoperative treatment, with historical studies showing an 80 to 92% failure rate.[53,54,55]
- Therefore, there is no role for nonoperative treatment in adults unless the patient is not a surgical candidate.

2. Open Reduction and Internal Fixation of the Radius

- Accomplished through modified Henry volar approach as described in the prior section on distal radius fractures.
- Fixation should include six cortices above and below the fracture utilizing a 3.5-mm plate.[60]

3. Distal Radioulnar Joint Reduction and Stabilization

- After fixation of the radius, the DRUJ should be tested intraoperatively for stability.

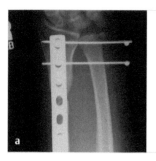
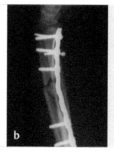

Fig. 8.6 (a, b) Pinning technique for an unstable distal radioulnar joint (DRUJ).

- If the DRUJ does not reduce with fixation of the radius, interposition of soft tissue, most commonly the ECU tendon, should be suspected. The joint should then be openly reduced.
- You may be able to feel the empty ECU tendon sheath on examination, termed the "empty sulcus sign."[65]
- An unstable, yet reduced, DRUJ can then be pinned with two parallel K-wires just proximal to the joint (▶ Fig. 8.6).

References

[1] Johnell O, Kanis JA. An estimate of the worldwide prevalence and disability associated with osteoporotic fractures. Osteoporos Int. 2006; 17(12):1726–1733

[2] Shauver MJ, Yin H,. Banerjee M, Chung KC. Current and future national costs to medicare for the treatment of distal radius fracture in the lderly. J Hand Surg Am. 2011; 36(8):1282–1287

[3] Cuddihy MT, Gabriel SE, Crowson CS, O'Fallon WM, Melton LJ, III. Forearm fractures as predictors of subsequent osteoporotic fractures. Osteoporos Int. 1999; 9(6):469–475

[4] Mallmin H, Ljunghall S, Persson I, Naessén T, Krusemo UB, Bergström R. Fracture of the distal forearm as a forecaster of subsequent hip fracture: a population-based cohort study with 24 years of follow-up. Calcif Tissue Int. 1993; 52(4):269–272

[5] Davis DI, Baratz M. Soft tissue complications of distal radius fractures. Hand Clin. 2010; 26(2):229–235

[6] Vance RM, Gelberman RH. Acute ulnar neuropathy with fractures at the wrist. J Bone Joint Surg Am. 1978; 60(7):962–965

[7] Ekrol I, Duckworth AD, Ralston SH, Court-Brown CM, McQueen MM. The influence of vitamin C on the outcome of distal radial fractures: a double-blind, randomized controlled trial. J Bone Joint Surg Am. 2014; 96 (17):1451–1459

[8] Medoff RJ. Essential radiographic evaluation for distal radius fractures. Hand Clin. 2005; 21(3):279–288

[9] Lafontaine M, Hardy D, Delince P. Stability assessment of distal radius fractures. Injury. 1989; 20(4):208–210

[10] Ilyas AM, Jupiter JB. Distal radius fractures—classification of treatment and indications for surgery. Orthop Clin North Am. 2007; 38(2):167–173, v

[11] The Treatment of Distal Radius Fractures, Guideline and Evidence Report. AAOS. https://www.aaos.org/globalassets/quality-and-practice-resources/distal-radius/distal-radius-fractures-clinical-practice-guideline.pdf Published December 5, 2009

[12] Shauver MJ, Clapham PJ, Chung KC. An economic analysis of outcomes and complications of treating distal radius fractures in the elderly. J Hand Surg Am. 2011; 36(12):1912–8.e1, 3

[13] Gelberman RH, Szabo RM, Mortensen WW. Carpal tunnel pressures and wrist position in patients with Colles' fractures. J Trauma. 1984; 24(8):747–749

[14] Trumble TE, Wagner W, Hanel DP, Vedder NB, Gilbert M. Intrafocal (Kapandji) pinning of distal radius fractures with and without external fixation. J Hand Surg Am. 1998; 23(3):381–394

[15] Agee JM. Application of multiplanar ligamentotaxis to external fixation of distal radius fractures. Iowa Orthop J. 1994; 14:31–37

[16] Hanel DP, Lu TS, Weil WM. Bridge plating of distal radius fractures: the Harborview method. Clin Orthop Relat Res. 2006; 445(445):91–99

[17] Burke EF, Singer RM. Treatment of comminuted distal radius with the use of an internal distraction plate. Tech Hand Up Extrem Surg. 1998; 2(4):248–252

[18] Orbay JL. The treatment of unstable distal radius fractures with volar fixation. Hand Surg. 2000; 5(2):103–112

[19] Rozental TD, Blazar PE, Franko OI, Chacko AT, Earp BE, Day CS. Functional outcomes for unstable distal radial fractures treated with open reduction and internal fixation or closed reduction and percutaneous fixation. A prospective randomized trial. J Bone Joint Surg Am. 2009; 91(8):1837–1846

[20] Ahsan ZS, Yao J. The importance of pronator quadratus repair in the treatment of distal radius fractures with volar plating. Hand (N Y). 2012; 7(3):276–280

[21] Agee JM. Distal radius fractures: multiplanar ligamentotaxis. Hand Clin. 1993; 9(4):577–585

[22] Wright TW, Horodyski M, Smith DW. Functional outcome of unstable distal radius fractures: ORIF with a volar fixed-angle tine plate versus external fixation. J Hand Surg Am. 2005; 30(2):289–299

[23] Benson LS, Minihane KP, Stern LD, Eller E, Seshadri R. The outcome of intra-articular distal radius fractures treated with fragment-specific fixation. J Hand Surg Am. 2006; 31(8):1333–1339

[24] Swigart CR, Wolfe SW. Limited incision open techniques for distal radius fracture management. Orthop Clin North Am. 2001; 32(2):317–327, ix

[25] Taylor KF, Parks BG, Segalman KA. Biomechanical stability of a fixed-angle volar plate versus fragment-specific fixation system: cyclic testing in a C2-type distal radius cadaver fracture model. J Hand Surg Am. 2006; 31(3):373–381

[26] Medoff RJ. Chapter 10: Fragment-Specific Fixation of Distal Radius Fractures. In: Operative Techniques in Orthopedic Surgery. 2nd ed. 2016;2627–2645

[27] Schumer ED, Leslie BM. Fragment-specific fixation of distal radius fractures using the Trimed device. Tech Hand Up Extrem Surg. 2005; 9(2):74–83

[28] Yu YR, Makhni MC, Tabrizi S, Rozental TD, Mundanthanam G, Day CS. Complications of low-profile dorsal versus volar locking plates in the distal radius: a comparative study. J Hand Surg Am. 2011; 36(7):1135–1141

[29] Rozental TD, Beredjiklian PK, Bozentka DJ. Functional outcome and complications following two types of dorsal plating for unstable fractures of the distal part of the radius. J Bone Joint Surg Am. 2003; 85(10):1956–1960

[30] Trease C, McIff T, Toby EB. Locking versus nonlocking T-plates for dorsal and volar fixation of dorsally comminuted distal radius fractures: a biomechanical study. J Hand Surg Am. 2005; 30(4):756–763

[31] Zollinger PE, Tuinebreijer WE, Breederveld RS, Kreis RW. Can vitamin C prevent complex regional pain syndrome in patients with wrist fractures? A randomized, controlled, multicenter dose-response study. J Bone Joint Surg Am. 2007; 89(7):1424–1431

[32] Evaniew N, McCarthy C, Kleinlugtenbelt YV, Ghert M, Bhandari M. Vitamin C to prevent complex regional pain syndrome in patients with distal radius fractures: a meta-analysis of randomized controlled trials. J Orthop Trauma. 2015; 29(8):e235–e241

[33] Malay S, Chung KC. Testing the validity of preventing chronic regional pain syndrome with vitamin C after distal radius fracture. [Corrected]. J Hand Surg Am. 2014; 39(11):2251–2257

[34] Meena S, Sharma P, Gangary SK, Chowdhury B. Role of vitamin C in prevention of complex regional pain syndrome after distal radius fractures: a meta-analysis. Eur J Orthop Surg Traumatol. 2015; 25(4):637–641

[35] Harness NG, Jupiter JB, Orbay JL, Raskin KB, Fernandez DL. Loss of fixation of the volar lunate facet fragment in fractures of the distal part of the radius. J Bone Joint Surg Am. 2004; 86(9):1900–1908

[36] Richards RS, Bennett JD, Roth JH, Milne K, Jr. Arthroscopic diagnosis of intra-articular soft tissue injuries associated with distal radial fractures. J Hand Surg Am. 1997; 22(5):772–776

[37] af Ekenstam F, Hagert CG. Anatomical studies on the geometry and stability of the distal radio ulnar joint. Scand J Plast Reconstr Surg. 1985; 19(1):17–25

[38] Arora R, Lutz M, Hennerbichler A, Krappinger D, Espen D, Gabl M. Complications following internal fixation of unstable distal radius fracture with a palmar locking-plate. J Orthop Trauma. 2007; 21(5):316–322

[39] Roth KM, Blazar PE, Earp BE, Han R, Leung A. Incidence of extensor pollicis longus tendon rupture after non-displaced distal radius fractures. J Hand Surg Am. 2012; 37(5):942–947

[40] Ozer K, Wolf JM, Watkins B, Hak DJ. Comparison of 4 fluoroscopic views for dorsal cortex screw penetration after volar plating of the distal radius. J Hand Surg Am. 2012; 37(5):963–967

[41] Soong M, Earp BE, Bishop G, Leung A, Blazar P. Volar locking plate implant prominence and flexor tendon rupture. J Bone Joint Surg Am. 2011; 93(4):328–335

[42] Casaletto JA, Machin D, Leung R, Brown DJ. Flexor pollicis longus tendon ruptures after palmar plate fixation of fractures of the distal radius. J Hand Surg Eur Vol. 2009; 34(4):471–474

[43] Wurtzel CNW, Burns GT, Zhu AF, Ozer K. Effects of volar tilt, wrist extension, and plate position on contact between flexor pollicis longus tendon and volar plate. J Hand Surg Am. 2017; 42(12):996–1001

[44] Dyer G, Lozano-Calderon S, Gannon C, Baratz M, Ring D. Predictors of acute carpal tunnel syndrome associated with fracture of the distal radius. J Hand Surg Am. 2008; 33(8):1309–1313

[45] Ward CM, Kuhl TL, Adams BD. Early complications of volar plating of distal radius fractures and their relationship to surgeon experience. Hand (N Y). 2011; 6(2):185–189

[46] Smith TO, Drew B, Toms AP, Jerosch-Herold C, Chojnowski AJ. Diagnostic accuracy of magnetic resonance imaging and magnetic resonance arthrography for triangular fibrocartilaginous complex injury: a systematic review and meta-analysis. J Bone Joint Surg Am. 2012; 94(9):824–832

[47] May MM, Lawton JN, Blazar PE. Ulnar styloid fractures associated with distal radius fractures: incidence and implications for distal radioulnar joint instability. J Hand Surg Am. 2002; 27(6):965–971

[48] Wijffels M, Ring D. The influence of non-union of the ulnar styloid on pain, wrist function and instability after distal radius fracture. J Hand Microsurg. 2011; 3(1):11–14

[49] Wysocki RW, Ruch DS. Ulnar styloid fracture with distal radius fracture. J Hand Surg Am. 2012; 37(3):568–569

[50] Botte MJ, Cohen MS, Lavernia CJ, von Schroeder HP, Gellman H, Zinberg EM. The dorsal branch of the ulnar nerve: an anatomic study. J Hand Surg Am. 1990; 15(4):603–607

[51] Cooper A. A Treatise on Dislocations and on Fractures of the Joints. 4th ed. London: Longman and Underwood; 1824:470–476

[52] Galeazzi R. Über ein besonderes Syndrom bei Verletzungen im Bereich der Unterarmknocken. Arch Orthop Unfallchir. 1934; 35:557–562

[53] Hughston JC. Fracture of the distal radial shaft; mistakes in management. J Bone Joint Surg Am. 1957; 39-A (2):249–264, passim

[54] Wong PC. Galeazzi fracture–dislocations in Singapore 1960–64; incidence and results of treatment. Singapore Med J. 1967; 8(3):186–193

[55] Mikić ZD. Galeazzi fracture-dislocations. J Bone Joint Surg Am. 1975; 57(8):1071–1080

[56] Stuart PR, Berger RA, Linscheid RL, An KN. The dorsopalmar stability of the distal radioulnar joint. J Hand Surg Am. 2000; 25(4):689–699

[57] Palmer AK, Werner FW. The triangular fibrocartilage complex of the wrist—anatomy and function. J Hand Surg Am. 1981; 6(2):153–162

[58] Rettig ME, Raskin KB. Galeazzi fracture-dislocation: a new treatment-oriented classification. J Hand Surg Am. 2001; 26(2):228–235

[59] Ring D, Rhim R, Carpenter C, Jupiter JB. Isolated radial shaft fractures are more common than Galeazzi fractures. J Hand Surg Am. 2006; 31(1):17–21

[60] Korompilias AV, Lykissas MG, Kostas-Agnantis IP, Beris AE, Soucacos PN. Distal radioulnar joint instability (Galeazzi type injury) after internal fixation in relation to the radius fracture pattern. J Hand Surg Am. 2011; 36(5):847–852

[61] Bruckner JD, Lichtman DM, Alexander AH. Complex dislocations of the distal radioulnar joint: recognition and management. Clin Orthop Relat Res. 1992(275):90–103

[62] Moore TM, Lester DK, Sarmiento A. The stabilizing effect of soft-tissue constraints in artificial Galeazzi fractures. Clin Orthop Relat Res. 1985(194):189–194

[63] Amrami KK, Moran SL, Berger RA, Ehman EC, Felmlee JP. Imaging the distal radioulnar joint. Hand Clin. 2010; 26(4):467–475

[64] Carlsen BT, Dennison DG, Moran SL. Acute dislocations of the distal radioulnar joint and distal ulna fractures. Hand Clin. 2010; 26(4):503–516

[65] Paley D, McMurtry RY, Murray JF. Dorsal dislocation of the ulnar styloid and extensor carpi ulnaris tendon into the distal radioulnar joint: the empty sulcus sign. J Hand Surg Am. 1987; 12(6):1029–1032

9 Triangular Fibrocartilage Complex and Distal Radioulnar Joint Pathology

Cory Lebowitz and Jonas L. Matzon

Abstract

The triangular fibrocartilage complex (TFCC) and distal radioulnar joint (DRUJ) are complex structures. This chapter provides details on the anatomy and function of these structures. Furthermore, it reviews the diagnosis and treatment of pathologies, such as TFCC tears, ulnar impaction syndrome, and DRUJ instability.

Keywords: Triangular fibrocartilage complex (TFCC), distal radioulnar joint (DRUJ), ulnar impaction syndrome, TFCC tears, DRUJ instability, arthroscopy

I. Introduction

A. Background

- The distal radioulnar joint (DRUJ) is an inherently unstable joint.
- The triangular fibrocartilage complex (TFCC) is a ligamentous structure that provides support to the DRUJ as well as several ulnocarpal articulations.

B. Epidemiology

- TFCC injury is a common cause of ulnar-sided wrist pain.
  - Evidence of torn TFCC is seen in 78% of distal radius fractures.[1]
  - As patients age, degenerative TFCC tears become nearly universal.[2]
- Traumatic TFCC injuries have the potential to cause DRUJ instability.

II. Anatomy and Function

A. Triangular Fibrocartilage Complex

- Radioulnar ligaments (RUL): Originate from the palmar and dorsal margins of the sigmoid notch to insert superficially at the ulnar styloid and deep at the fovea (▶ Fig. 9.1).
  - Function: Primary stabilizers of the DRUJ.
  - The ligamentum subcruentum is the tissue between the superficial and deep insertions of the RUL.
- Articular disk: Avascular, triangular-shaped fibrocartilage that attaches radially at the sigmoid notch of the radius and then blends peripherally to the RUL.
  - Function: Transmits and absorbs compressive forces through the wrist.
- Meniscal homologue (MH): Fibrous tissue that adds to the hammock-like shape of the distal portion of the TFCC between the ulnar capsule, disk, and triquetrum.
- Ulnocarpal ligaments: Volar structures that include the ulnolunate, ulnotriquetral, and ulnocapitate ligaments.
- Extensor carpi ulnar (ECU) sheath: Reinforces the dorsal capsule.

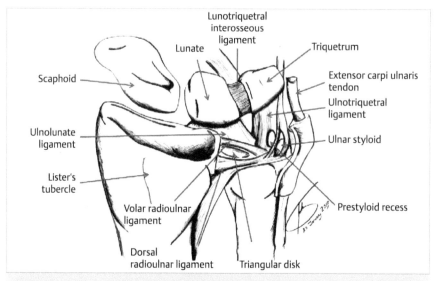

Fig. 9.1 Illustration of the major components of the triangular fibrocartilage complex and distal radioulnar joint. The primary stabilizer of the distal radioulnar joint is the triangular fibrocartilage complex. Used with permission of Mespreuve et al.[3]

B. Distal Radioulnar Joint

- Osseous anatomy is responsible for 20% of joint stability.[4]
  - Sigmoid notch is concave with a large radius of curvature to support the convex ulnar head and to allow for controlled pronation and supination.
- Soft-tissue anatomy is responsible for 80% of joint stability.[4]
  - Palmar and dorsal RUL (see above).
  - The ECU and pronator quadratus (PQ) dynamically stabilize the distal ulna and DRUJ.
  - The distal interosseous membrane (IOM) restricts movement of the radius during forearm rotation.
- Function: Allows forearm rotation and transmits forces across the wrist.

III. Diagnosis

A. History

- Ulnar-sided wrist pain
  - Traumatic onset: Classic mechanism is falling on an outstretched, pronated arm.
  - Atraumatic onset: Pain that worsens with pronation/supination and/or power grip.

B. Physical Examination

- Inspection for any deformity, swelling, and/or asymmetry.
- Active and passive wrist range of motion focusing on pronation and supination.

- Provocative maneuvers:
  - Foveal sign: Tenderness to palpation at the fovea, which is the soft spot between the ECU and flexor carpi ulnaris (FCU), proximal to the pisiform and just distal to the ulnar styloid.
    - 95.2% sensitivity and 86.5% specificity for TFCC tear.[5]
  - Ulnocarpal stress test: Pain with ulnar deviation and forearm rotation.
    - Sensitive for ulnar impaction syndrome, but not specific.
  - Shuck test: Performed by stabilizing the radius and translating the ulna in full supination, pronation, and neutral while comparing with contralateral extremity.
    - Used to assess DRUJ stability.
  - Press test: Patient uses the arms of a chair to rise from a seated position, which in turn creates dynamic loading.
    - The sensitivity of detecting TFCC lesions is up to 100%.[6]

C. Diagnostic Imaging

- Radiographs: Posteroanterior (PA), lateral, and oblique
  - Assess for ulnar variance, alignment, fractures, and degenerative changes:
    - PA may show lesions on the lunate, triquetrum, or ulnar head in the setting of impaction syndrome.
    - Lateral can be helpful in diagnosing DRUJ instability.
- Dynamic computed tomography
  - Bilateral DRUJ in pronation, neutral, and supination to evaluate subtle instability.
- Magnetic resonance imaging (MRI) (▶ Fig. 9.2)
  - Full-thickness TFCC tears: 75% sensitivity and 81% specificity.[7]

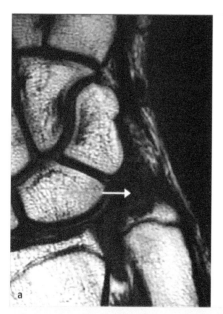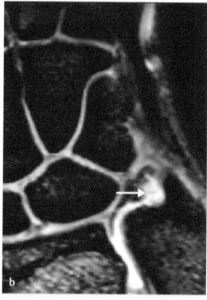

Fig. 9.2 Magnetic resonance imaging (MRI) of a triangular fibrocartilage complex (TFCC) 1B tear (*arrow*) on coronal T1–WI **(a)** and coronal FS T2–WI **(b)**. Used with permission of Mespreuve et al.[3]

Table 9.1 Palmer classification of triangular fibrocartilage complex (TFCC) tears

Class	Description
Class 1	Acute traumatic
Type 1A	Central perforation
Type 1B	Peripheral ulnar avulsion, with or without distal ulnar fracture
Type 1C	Distal avulsion
Type 1D	Radial avulsion, with or without sigmoid notch fracture
Class 2	Degenerative
Type 2A	TFCC wear
Type 2B	Type 2A + lunate and/or ulnar chondromalacia
Type 2C	TFCC perforation with lunate and/or ulnar chondromalacia
Type 2D	Type 2C + lunotriquetral ligament perforation
Type 2E	Type 2D + ulnocarpal arthritis

- MRI arthrograms
  - Full-thickness TFCC tears: 84% sensitivity and 95% specificity.[7]
- Arthroscopy
  - Considered gold standard for TFCC tears:
    - However, inter- and intraobserver reliability of TFCC tear is only 66.7 and 67.4%, respectively.[8]
  - Provocative maneuvers:
    - Trampoline test: Positive when the TFCC is soft and compliant when probed.
    - Hook test: Foveal disruption suspected when the TFCC can be pulled radially and upward toward the center of the radiocarpal joint with a probe.

IV. TFCC Tears and Ulnar Impaction Syndrome

A. Classification

- Palmer classification (▶ Table 9.1)
  - Class 1: Traumatic
    - Class 1A is most common with a low risk of DRUJ instability.[5]
    - Classes 1B–1D should be suspected with a positive trampoline test.
    - Class 1C is less common and can be in combination with 1B.
    - Class 1D frequently accompanies a displaced distal radius fracture.
  - Class 2: Degenerative (ulnar impaction syndrome)
    - Result from chronic loading through the ulnocarpal joint.

B. Nonoperative Treatment

- Indications: Initial treatment for all TFCC tears in the absence of DRUJ instability.
- Options include activity modification, immobilization, nonsteroidal anti-inflammatory drugs (NSAIDs), and corticosteroid injections.

C. Operative Treatment

1. Indications

- Failure of nonoperative management with persistent symptoms and/or DRUJ instability.

2. Options

- Arthroscopic debridement
  - Indications: Class 1A tears.
  - Technique: Preserve 1 to 2 mm of the peripheral articular disk to preserve RUL and to retain kinematics.
- Arthroscopic or open repair
  - Indications: Class1B/1C/1D tears.
  - Techniques:
    - Repair to ulnar capsule with inside-out, outside-in, or all-arthroscopic technique.
    - Transosseous sutures or bone anchors to restore the tissue back to the fovea or distal radius.
- TFCC reconstruction
  - Indications: Persistent DRUJ instability following primary TFCC repair.
  - Techniques:
    - Direct radioulnar tether that is extrinsic to the joint.
    - Indirect radioulnar link through tenodesis or an ulnocarpal sling.
    - Reconstruction of RUL with intra-articular tendon graft.
  - Wafer procedure
    - Indications: Class 2 degenerative tears in the setting of ulnar positive wrist.
    - Technique: Open or arthroscopic partial resection of the distal ulna that maintains DRUJ stability while avoiding need for hardware.
  - Ulnar shortening osteotomy
    - Indications: Class 2 tears in the setting of ulnar positive variance.
    - Techniques: Shortening through diaphysis or metaphysis retains entire cartilaginous surface of the distal ulna while theoretically tightening the ulnocarpal ligaments (and the DRUJ).

V. DRUJ Instability

A. Fractures with DRUJ Instability

- Galeazzi fractures: Radial fractures at the junction of the middle and distal third.
  - Considered "fracture of necessity" secondary to poor results without operative intervention and high association with DRUJ instability.
  - Incidence of DRUJ instability is based on fracture location:[9]
    - 55% when fracture is within 7.5 cm of the mid-articular surface.
    - 6% when fracture is greater than 7.5 cm from mid-articular surface.
  - Treatment: Radius open reduction internal fixation (ORIF).
  - If the DRUJ remains stable after fixation, early motion can be initiated.
  - If there is instability after fixation, options include:
    - Immobilization in supination for 4 to 6 weeks.
    - Acute TFCC repair.

- Essex-Lopresti injury: Radial head fracture with interosseous ligament disruption.
  - Treatment: Radial head ORIF or arthroplasty with immobilization in supination, acute TFCC repair, or interosseous ligament reconstruction.
  - Results: Often dependent upon recognition.

B. Distal Radius Malunions

- Malunions change the normal axis of rotation, reduce joint incongruity, stress the TFCC, and limit forearm pronation-supination.
  - Dramatic incongruency of the DRUJ when the dorsal tilt exceeds 10 degrees.[10]
- Treatment: Extra-articular osteotomy to restore the sigmoid notch's orientation and DRUJ stability.

C. Simple Dislocations

- Isolated DRUJ instability is relatively uncommon:
  - Dorsal dislocations: Most common and usually secondary to fall on an outstretched hand with the wrist in hyperpronation and extension.
  - Volar dislocations: Typically due to an axial load to a hypersupinated forearm or a direct blow to the ulna.
- Treatment:
  - Closed reduction with immobilization in position of stability for 4 to 6 weeks:
    - Dorsal dislocations are typically stable in supination.
    - Palmar dislocations are usually stable in pronation.
  - Radioulnar pinning in the stable position or TFCC repair/reconstruction:
    - When stability only occurs in extreme supination or pronation.

References

[1] Lindau T, Arner M, Hagberg L. Intraarticular lesions in distal fractures of the radius in young adults: a descriptive arthroscopic study in 50 patients. J Hand Surg [Br]. 1997; 22(5):638–643

[2] Mikić ZD. Age changes in the triangular fibrocartilage of the wrist joint. J Anat. 1978; 126(Pt 2):367–384

[3] Mespreuve M, Vanhoenacker F, Verstraete K. Correction: imaging findings of the distal radio-ulnar joint in trauma. J Belg Soc Radiol. 2015; 99(1):129–130

[4] Zimmerman RM, Jupiter JB. Instability of the distal radioulnar joint. J Hand Surg Eur Vol. 2014; 39(7):727–738

[5] Pidgeon TS, Waryasz G, Carnevale J, DaSilva MF. Triangular fibrocartilage complex: an anatomic review. JBJS Rev. 2015; 3(1):1

[6] Lester B, Halbrecht J, Levy IM, Gaudinez R. "Press test" for office diagnosis of triangular fibrocartilage complex tears of the wrist. Ann Plast Surg. 1995; 35(1):41–45

[7] Smith TO, Drew B, Toms AP, Jerosch-Herold C, Chojnowski AJ. Diagnostic accuracy of magnetic resonance imaging and magnetic resonance arthrography for triangular fibrocartilaginous complex injury: a systematic review and meta-analysis. J Bone Joint Surg Am. 2012; 94(9):824–832

[8] Park A, Lutsky K, Matzon J, Leinberry C, Chapman T, Beredjiklian PK. An evaluation of the reliability of wrist arthroscopy in the assessment of tears of the triangular fibrocartilage complex. J Hand Surg Am. 2018; 43(6):545–549

[9] Rettig ME, Raskin KB. Galeazzi fracture-dislocation: a new treatment-oriented classification. J Hand Surg Am. 2001; 26(2):228–235

[10] Kihara H, Palmer AK, Werner FW, Short WH, Fortino MD. The effect of dorsally angulated distal radius fractures on distal radioulnar joint congruency and forearm rotation. J Hand Surg Am. 1996; 21(1):40–47

10 Osteoarthritis of the Wrist and Hand

Brittany Homcha and Kenneth F. Taylor

Abstract

Osteoarthritis of the wrist and hand involves progressive destruction of articular carti-lage and associated subchondral bony changes including sclerosis, cystic degeneration, and osteophyte formation. Inflammation is not a significant aspect of this process. Onset is often insidious in nature and thought to be age and wear related. Initial treat-ment modalities include patient education, joint preservation, splint wear, and other physical modalities including therapy, corticosteroid injection, and nonsteroidal anti-inflammatory medications. Surgical options include osteotomy, soft tissue interposi-tion, joint arthrodesis, and arthroplasty.

Keywords: Osteoarthritis, hand, wrist, joint, arthrodesis, arthroplasty

I. Distal Interphalangeal Joint

A. Background

- Highest prevalence of osteoarthritis (OA) in the hand;[1] commonly accompanied by Heberden's nodes and mucus cysts (▶ Fig. 10.1 and ▶ Fig. 10.2).

B. Surgical Treatment

- Mucous cyst excision: Osteophytes must be excised or mucus cysts will recur.
- Arthrodesis: Biomechanical studies demonstrate comparative performance between K-wire fixation (parallel or crossed) and compression screw fixation.[2]
  - Union rates for headless compression screw approaches 94% (▶ Fig. 10.3 and ▶ Fig. 10.4).[3]

II. Proximal Interphalangeal Joint

A. Background

- More common in women; favors dominant hand; accompanied by Bouchard's nodes.

B. Appearance

- May be erosive or nonerosive with abrupt symptom onset of pain, erythema, and loss of joint function along with instability more common with the former; indolent onset more frequently encountered with nonerosive.

C. Radiographs

- Central joint degeneration and edge proliferation suggestive of erosive arthritis (▶ Fig. 10.5 and ▶ Fig. 10.6).

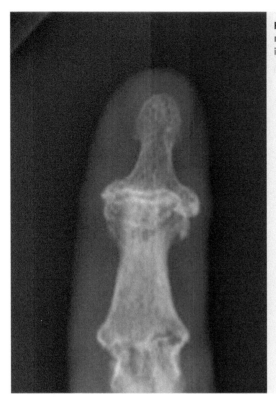

Fig. 10.1 Posteroanterior (PA) radiograph demonstrating distal interphalangeal joint osteoarthritis.

D. Conservative Treatment

• Patient education, anti-inflammatory medications, injection.

E. Surgical Treatment

• Arthrodesis: Degree of flexion increases from radial to ulnar (40–55 degrees).
• Arthroplasty: Multiple material options exist for arthroplasty including silicone, pyrocarbon, and metal-polyethylene.

III. Metacarpophalangeal Joint

A. Background

• Less common in OA; thumb metacarpophalangeal (MCP) arthritis may be associated with carpometacarpal (CMC) joint arthritis.

B. Surgical Treatment

• Arthrodesis; arthroplasty (silicone, nonconstrained pyrocarbon, or metal-polyethylene).

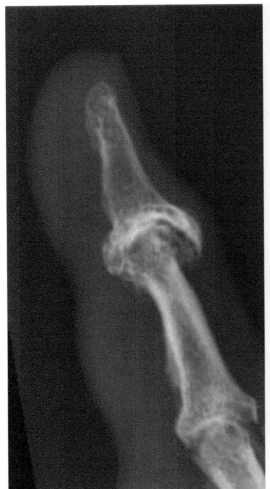

Fig. 10.2 Lateral radiograph demonstrating distal interphalangeal joint osteoarthritis.

IV. Trapeziometacarpal/Thumb CMC/Basilar Joint Arthritis

A. Epidemiology

- Affects women more frequently than men, often in later decades of life at up to 36% of postmenopausal women.[4]

B. Physical Examination

- Pain or crepitus with axial grind test (axial compression and circumduction while stabilizing surrounding joints).
- Progressive "zig zag" deformity—metacarpal adduction, MCP hyperextension, and first web space contracture.

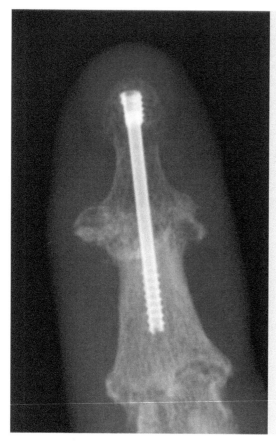

Fig. 10.3 Posteroanterior (PA) radiograph of distal interphalangeal joint arthrodesis with headless compression screw.

C. Radiographic Examination

- Include true anteroposterior (AP) (Robert's view): Forearm in maximal pronation with dorsum of thumb resting on cassette.
- Eaton-Littler classification: Classically used but poor/fair interobserver reliability.[5]
  - I: Normal joint contour, no joint space narrowing or sclerosis, mild joint space widening (synovitis).
  - II: Mild joint space narrowing, mild sclerosis with or without subchondral cysts, <2 mm osteophytes.
  - III: Substantial joint space narrowing, marked sclerosis with or without subchondral cysts, >2 mm osteophytes.
  - IV: Pantrapezial arthritis (scaphotrapeziotrapezoid [STT] joint involvement).

D. Management

1. Conservative

- Splinting—no consensus on optimal brace type.
- Corticosteroid injection—intra-articular.

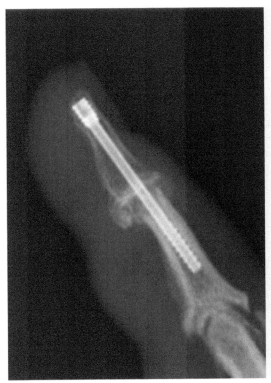

Fig. 10.4 Lateral radiograph of distal interphalangeal joint arthrodesis with headless compression screw.

2. Surgical

- Must recognize potential involvement of STT joint.
- Arthrodesis in 20 degrees radial abduction and 40 degrees of palmar abduction for young laborers.
- Trapeziectomy with or without tendon suspensionplasty (slip abductor pollicis longus [APL], flexor carpi radialis [FCR], extensor carpi radialis longus [ECRL]).
- Trapeziectomy and suture suspension device.

V. Scaphotrapeziotrapezoid (STT) Joint

A. Surgical Treatment Options

- Trapeziectomy with trapezoid osteotomy (▶ Fig. 10.7).
- STT arthrodesis: 75% motion of normal wrist, high nonunion rate.[6]
- Distal pole scaphoid excision: Must ensure absence of midcarpal instability.[7]

VI. Pisotriquetral Joint

A. Surgical Treatment Options

- Excision of pisiform.
- Pisotriquetral arthrodesis.

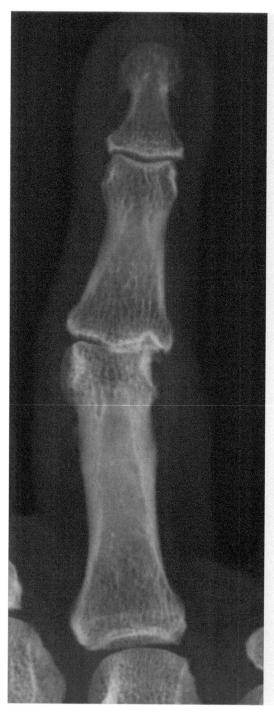

Fig. 10.5 Posteroanterior (PA) radiograph demonstrating proximal interphalangeal joint osteoarthritis.

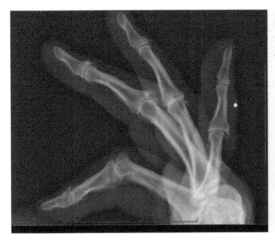

Fig. 10.6 Lateral radiograph demonstrating proximal interphalangeal joint osteoarthritis.

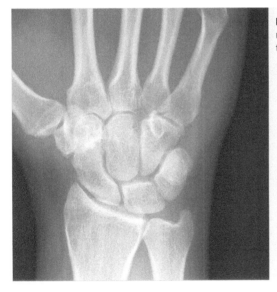

Fig. 10.7 Posteroanterior (PA) radiograph demonstrating scaphotrapeziotrapezoid arthritis.

VII. Radiocarpal Arthritis

A. Overview

- Multiple etiologies including traumatic (scaphoid nonunion advanced collapse [SNAC] and scapholunate advanced collapse [SLAC]), idiopathic, avascular (Kienbock's disease and Preiser's disease), congenital (Madelung's deformity).

B. Physical Examination

- Palpation of wrist structures with attention to radiocarpal, ulnocarpal, DRUJ, and intercarpal joints.
- Diagnostic and prognostic cortisone or anesthetic injections may be helpful adjunct.

C. Radiographic Examination

- Evaluate adjacent joints as these influence treatment choice and outcome (▶ Fig. 10.8).

D. Surgical Management

- Partial wrist denervation
  - ○ Anterior interosseous nerve (AIN) and posterior interosseous nerve (PIN) neurectomy from single incision.
  - ○ Benefits: Pain relief without loss of proprioception, stiffness, immobilization, and significant recovery time; does not preclude later bony procedures.[8]
  - ○ AIN innervates volar wrist periosteum at capsule and ligament insertions, and PIN innervates central two-thirds of wrist.
    - – Preoperative nerve block may not be predictive of relief with neurectomy.[9]
- Proximal row carpectomy (PRC) (▶ Fig. 10.9)
  - ○ Benefits: Technically less demanding, no requirement for postoperative union leading to decreased postoperative immobilization, may have increased ROM compared to four corner fusion although slightly lower grip strength.[10]
  - ○ Contraindications: Capitate arthritis (will become load-bearing joint with radius).

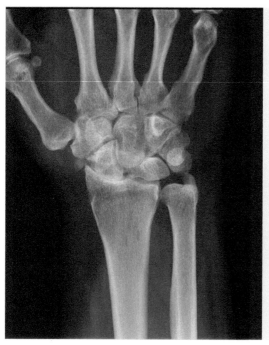

Fig. 10.8 Posteroanterior (PA) radiograph demonstrating radiocarpal arthritis.

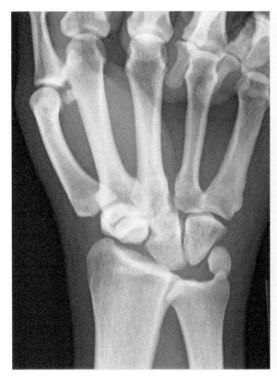

Fig. 10.9 Posteroanterior (PA) radiograph demonstrating proximal row carpectomy.

- Four corner arthrodesis (▶ Fig. 10.10)
  - Benefits: Preserve carpal height, improved grip strength relative to PRC.
  - Alternative modification: Three corner arthrodesis with scaphoidectomy and triquetrum excision also an option with slightly lower grip strength (72 vs. 94%) and increased ROM (70 vs. 64%) of contralateral side compared to four corner arthrodesis.[11]
- Radiocarpal arthrodesis: Radioscapholunate, radiolunate; preserves midcarpal joint motion.
- Total wrist arthrodesis: Usually in slight extension; preserves grip and forearm rotation (▶ Fig. 10.11).
- Arthroplasty
  - Typically performed on rheumatoid patients; survival rates at 5 years; vary from 57 to 100% with complication rate of up to 68% (range 11–68.7%).[12]
  - Careful patient selection required; however, results were not superior to total wrist arthrodesis.

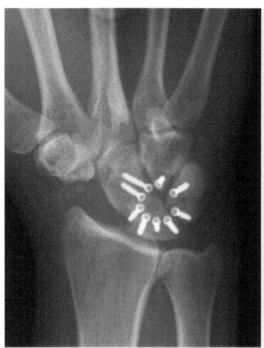

Fig. 10.10 Posteroanterior (PA) radiograph demonstrating scaphoidectomy and four corner arthrodesis.

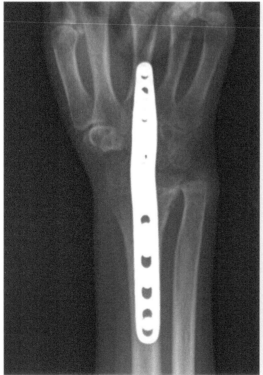

Fig. 10.11 Posteroanterior (PA) radiograph demonstrating wrist arthrodesis.

References

[1] Kaufmann RA, Lögters TT, Verbruggen G, Windolf J, Goitz RJ. Osteoarthritis of the distal interphalangeal joint. J Hand Surg Am. 2010; 35(12):2117–2125

[2] Rigot SK, Diaz-Garcia R, Debski RE, Fowler J. Biomechanical analysis of internal fixation methods for distal interphalangeal joint arthrodesis. Hand (N Y). 2016; 11(2):221–226

[3] Cox C, Earp BE, Floyd WE, IV, Blazar PE. Arthrodesis of the thumb interphalangeal joint and finger distal interphalangeal joints with a headless compression screw. J Hand Surg Am. 2014; 39(1):24–28

[4] Spaans AJ, van Minnen LP, Kon M, Schuurman AH, Schreuders AR, Vermeulen GM. Conservative treatment of thumb base osteoarthritis: a systematic review. J Hand Surg Am. 2015; 40(1):16–21.e1, 6

[5] Berger AJ, Momeni A, Ladd AL. Intra- and interobserver reliability of the Eaton classification for trapeziometacarpal arthritis: a systematic review. Clin Orthop Relat Res. 2014; 472(4):1155–1159

[6] Deans VM, Naqui Z, Muir LT. Scaphotrapeziotrapezoidal joint osteoarthritis: a systematic review of surgical treatment. J Hand Surg Asian Pac Vol. 2017; 22(1):1–9

[7] Garcia-Elias M, Lluch A. Partial excision of scaphoid: is it ever indicated? Hand Clin. 2001; 17(4):687–695, x

[8] Milone MT, Klifto CS, Catalano LW, III. Partial wrist denervation: the evidence behind a small fix for big problems. J Hand Surg Am. 2018; 43(3):272–277

[9] Storey PA, Lindau T, Jansen V, Woodbridge S, Bainbridge LC, Burke FD. Wrist denervation in isolation: a prospective outcome study with patient selection by wrist blockade. Hand Surg. 2011; 16(3):251–257

[10] Saltzman BM, Frank JM, Slikker W, Fernandez JJ, Cohen MS, Wysocki RW. Clinical outcomes of proximal row carpectomy versus four-corner arthrodesis for post-traumatic wrist arthropathy: a systematic review. J Hand Surg Eur Vol. 2015; 40(5):450–457

[11] Delattre O, Goulon G, Vogels J, Wavreille G, Lasnier A. Three-corner arthrodesis with scaphoid and triquetrum excision for wrist arthritis. J Hand Surg Am. 2015; 40(11):2176–2182

[12] Yeoh D, Tourret L. Total wrist arthroplasty: a systematic review of the evidence from the last 5 years. J Hand Surg Eur Vol. 2015; 40(5):458–468

11 Rheumatoid Arthritis and Other Inflammatory Arthropathies

Laura Lewallen, Hannah C. Langdell, and Scott D. Lifchez

Abstract

This chapter describes the symptoms, clinical and radiographic findings, as well as treatment options for rheumatoid arthritis and other inflammatory arthropathies.

Keywords: Rheumatoid arthritis, inflammatory arthritis, scleroderma, psoriasis, systemic lupus erythematosus

I. Rheumatoid Arthritis

A. Clinical Stages

- Stage 1: Synovial membrane inflammation and swelling without deformity.
- Stage 2: Cartilage damage and deformity that is passively correctable.
- Stage 3: Muscle atrophy and fixed deformity.
- Stage 4: Cessation of inflammatory process, formation of fibrous tissue, and/or bony fusion.

B. History and Physical Examination

1. History/Presentation

- Morning stiffness in the joints.
- Inability to extend the fingers.
- Inability to make a full fist with swan neck deformity.
- Involvement of multiple joints (usually the hands and feet) with relative sparing of distal interphalangeal (DIP) joints.
- Wrist weakness and pain worsened by forearm rotation.
- Common questions:
  - Prior rheumatologic diagnosis.
  - Duration of symptoms.
  - Type of onset (acute or insidious).
  - Other involved joints.
  - Medications for arthritis.
  - Ability to perform activities of daily living.

2. Physical Examination

- Hand
  - Soft tissue swelling of proximal interphalangeal (PIP) and metacarpophalangeal (CMC) joints.
  - Volar subluxation of proximal phalanges.
  - Ulnar drift of fingers (at MCP joints).
  - Chronic synovitis leading to tendon ruptures.

- Tendon sheath involvement—dorsal and volar aspects of wrist, volar surface of digits.
- Intra-articular involvement.
  - Boutonniere deformity—flexed PIP joints and extended DIP joints with elongation or rupture of central slip.
  - Swan neck deformity—PIP hyperextension, DIP flexion with dorsal subluxation of lateral bands.
  - Subcutaneous rheumatoid nodules[1]—olecranon, extensor surface of forearms, dorsal aspect of hands, and palmar aspect of digits.
  - Sudden loss of finger extension or flexion indicates rupture, which typically progresses from ulnar to radial.
    - Differential diagnosis for tendon rupture—MCP joint dislocation, displacement of extensor tendons into valleys between metacarpal heads (sagittal band rupture), posterior interosseous nerve compression leading to paralysis of the common extensor muscle.[2]
- Wrist
  - Ulnar styloid, ulnar head, and scaphoid are often first to develop synovitis.
  - Caput ulna syndrome:[3]
    - Destruction of ligamentous components leading to dorsal prominence of the distal ulna due to volar subluxation of the radius.
    - Volar subluxation of extensor carpi ulnaris (ECU).
    - Distal radial ulnar joint (DRUJ) instability.
    - Limited wrist dorsiflexion.
    - Radial deviation of wrist.
    - Risk of attrition or rupture of extensor digitorum communis (EDC) to small finger with or without ring finger.
  - Scaphoid instability.
  - Severe disease—volar dislocation of wrist, destruction of carpal bones, and radioulnar joint dissociation.
  - Mannerfelt syndrome[4]
    - Scaphoid osteophytes in the carpal tunnel leading to attritional flexor pollicis longus (FPL) ruptures.
    - Weak or absent flexion of the thumb distal phalanx.
    - Treatment involves spur excision in addition to tendon transfer or graft.

C. Imaging

- Plain posteroanterior (PA) and lateral radiographs:
  - Periarticular erosions.
  - Joint space narrowing.
  - Osteopenia in hand and wrist joints.

D. Management

1. Nonsurgical

- Medical
  - Nonsteroidal anti-inflammatory drugs (NSAIDs).
  - Corticosteroids.

- Nonbiologic disease modifying antirheumatic drugs (DMARDs)—methotrexate, leflunomide, sulfasalazine, and hydroxychloroquine.
- Biologic DMARDs—TNF-α and IL-1 inhibitors (infliximab, etanercept, and adalimumab).
- No consensus on when to hold DMARDs in perioperative period.[5]
- General recommendation is to hold for half-life of medication both preoperatively and postoperatively.
- Hold biologic 1 week before and after surgery.
- It is advisable to continue methotrexate postoperatively.
- Splinting[6]
  - PIP joint splint for mild Boutonniere deformity.
  - Working wrist splints.
  - Ulnar deviation splints.
  - Ring splint for swan neck deformity.
- Hand therapy.[7]

2. Surgical: Hand

- Rheumatoid nodules—excise if symptomatic.
- Tenosynovitis—intra-tendon nodules may cause triggering, treat with tenosynovectomy preferably before tendon ruptures.[8]
- Tendon ruptures[9,10]: Extensor ruptures most common, proceeds from ulnar to radial:
  - Due to attrition at distal ulna, Lister's tubercle, or scaphoid or due to tendon invasion by tenosynovium.
  - Extensor pollics longus (EPL) rupture:
    - Tendon transfers using extensor indicis proprius (EIP) (preferred), extensor carpi radialis longus (ECRL), or extensor digiti minimi (EDM).
    - Tendon grafting.
  - Finger extensor rupture
    - Direct repair.
    - Suture distal stump to adjacent extensor.
    - Tendon grafting from palmaris longus, ECRL, or extensor carpi radialis brevis (ECRB).
    - Tendon transfer using EIP to extensor digiti quinti (EDQ) for single small finger extensor rupture.
    - Tendon transfers using EIP for double ruptures.
    - Tendon transfers using flexor digitorum superficialis (FDS) for triple ruptures.
  - FPL rupture
    - Most common flexor tendon rupture.
    - Tendon graft—palmaris longus, slip of flexor carpi radialis (FCR) or abductor pollicis longus (APL).
    - Tendon transfer—ring finger FDS.
  - Flexor digitorum profundus (FDP) rupture
    - Palm or wrist level—suture distal tendon to adjacent tendon.
    - Remove diseased synovium from intact superficial flexor.
  - FDS rupture
    - Suture to adjacent tendons.
    - Tenosynovectomy to protect FDP tendons.

- ○ FDP and FDS rupture
  - – Suture to adjacent tendons.
  - – Bridge graft to reconstruct FDP using FDS.
  - – Fuse DIP and PIP joints.
  - ○ Synovectomy and removal of bone spurs as part of surgery for any rupture.
- Sagittal band ruptures
  - ○ May lead to subluxation or dislocation of extensor tendon.
  - ○ Radial band most common.
  - ○ Present with pain when extending MCP joint against resistance and pseudotriggering.
  - ○ Treatment
    - – Extension splinting for acute injuries.
    - – Direct repair.
    - – Reconstruction using strips of EDC or lumbrical transfer to EDC.
- MCP joint deformity
  - ○ Arthroplasty—silicone is standard.[11]
  - ○ Extensor tendon centralization.
  - ○ Radial collateral ligament repair.
- PIP joint deformity
  - ○ Boutonniere deformity—synovectomy, extensor reconstruction, fusion, and/or arthroplasty.
  - ○ Joints are generally surgically addressed in a proximal to distal direction (e.g., correct wrist before fingers).

3. Surgical: Wrist

- Preventative
  - ○ Synovectomy of radioulnar and radiocarpal joints.[12]
  - ○ Tenosynovectomy.
  - ○ Balancing of wrist extensors.
- Reconstructive
  - ○ DRUJ disease
    - – Darrach's procedure[13]—distal ulnar resection; use ECU for stabilization (▶ Fig. 11.1).
    - – Sauvé-Kapandji procedure[14]—radioulnar joint arthrodesis and the creation of a pseudoarthrosis proximal to the fusion; use pronator quadratus interposition for stabilization (▶ Fig. 11.2).
  - ○ Ulnocarpal ligamentous complex reconstruction.
  - ○ Radiocarpal joint arthroplasty.
  - ○ Partial wrist fusion.
  - ○ Total wrist arthrodesis (▶ Fig. 11.3).[15]

II. Scleroderma

A. Presentation

- Disorder of small blood vessels and connective tissues leading to fibrosis.
- Heart, lungs, kidney, and gastrointestinal tract involvement.
- Skin—fibrosis of face and hands.

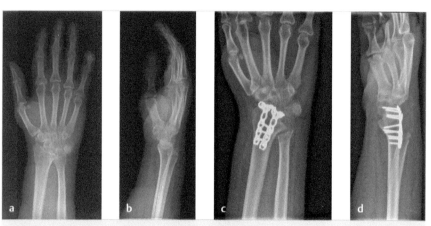

Fig. 11.1 Darrach and partial wrist arthrodesis (radioscapholunate). **(a, b)** Pre-op. **(c, d)** Post-op.

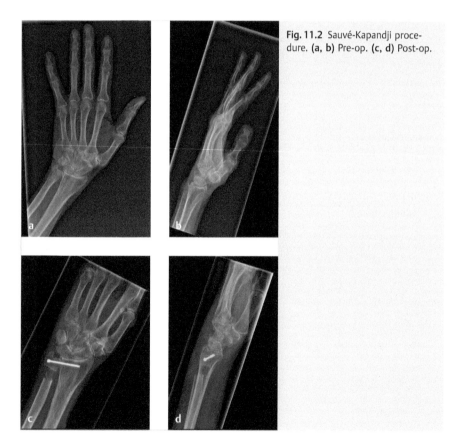

Fig. 11.2 Sauvé-Kapandji procedure. **(a, b)** Pre-op. **(c, d)** Post-op.

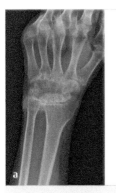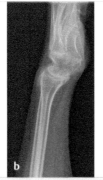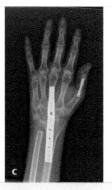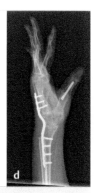

Fig. 11.3 Wrist arthrodesis with distal ulnar resection. **(a, b)** Pre-op. **(c, d)** Post-op.

- CREST syndrome—a type of limited scleroderma:
  - Calcinosis.
  - Raynaud's phenomenon.
  - Esophageal dysmotility.
  - Sclerodactyly.
  - Telangiectasias.
- Hand involvement—more common in patients with diffuse type of scleroderma.
  - Fibrosis leads to characteristic claw deformity and loss of function.
  - Raynaud's disease:[16]
    - Reduced digital circulation.
    - Skin ulcers: Open wounds can progress to osteomyelitis.
    - Gangrene.
    - Amputations.
  - Calcinosis—more common in limited cutaneous type.
  - PIP flexion contractures with MCP joint compensatory hyperextension.
  - Rupture of extension mechanism.

B. Imaging

- Plain PA and lateral radiographs
  - Acro-osteolysis—resorption of distal phalanx, most commonly the distal tuft.
  - Joint space narrowing.
  - Erosions.
  - Calcinosis—normally relatively diffuse, not discrete calcium deposit(s).
  - Resorption of the CMC joint with radial subluxation.

C. Management

1. Nonsurgical Measures

- Splinting, wound care, and topical antibiotics for ulcers.[17]
- Medications for ischemic manifestations: Calcium channel blockers,[18] particularly nifedipine, angiotensin-II receptor blockers, phosphodiesterase-5 (PDE-5) inhibitors,[19] and prostacyclin analogues.

2. Surgery

- Compromised wound healing due to poor circulation.
- Resection of bony prominence may be necessary to heal an open wound over MCP or PIP joints.
- Excision and irrigation for symptomatic calcinosis.
- DIP joint fusion or amputation.
- PIP joint fusion or arthroplasty for fixed flexion contracture;[20] minimize hardware implanted.
- MCP joint resection arthroplasty for fixed hyperextension.[21]
- First web space deepening.
- Vascular insufficiency.
  - Sympathectomy:[22,23] Microscopically stripping the arterial adventitia or chemical sympathectomy utilizing botulinum toxin A.[24]
  - Interposition vein grafts to superficial palmar arch.

III. Psoriatic Arthritis

A. Presentation

- Seronegative spondyloarthropathy found in approximately 5% of patients with psoriasis.
- Asymmetric involvement of the hands.
- 25% have polyarthritis.
- 5% have DIP joint disease with erosion of terminal phalanges, nail pitting, and onycholysis.
- Digital deformity
  - Spontaneous ankyloses—DIP or PIP joints.
  - Osteolysis—bone destruction and joint space widening most commonly in DIP joints.
  - Swelling due to periosteum or tendon swelling.
  - Flexion deformity of PIP joints.
  - MCP joint extension contracture.
  - Arthritis mutilans—loss of bone with collapse and shortening of digit.[25]
- Thumb involvement
  - Stiffness at CMC joint.

B. Imaging

- Plain PA and lateral radiographs[26]
  - "Pencil-in-cup" deformity—tapering of proximal bone with distal bone. This includes destruction of the head of the middle phalanx and expansion of the base of the distal phalanx, creating a "pencil-in-cup" appearance.
  - "Opera-glass hand" deformity—collapse of the digits.
  - Fluffy periostitis due to periosteal calcification.

C. Management

1. Nonsurgical

- NSAIDs.[27]
- Intra-articular injections.
- DMARDs.

2. Surgical

- Fusion of PIP joint.
- Arthroplasty for MCP joint extension contracture.
- Early fusion and bone grafting for arthritis mutilans.
- Wrist fusion.
- Darrach's procedure—resection of distal ulna.

IV. Systemic Lupus Erythematosus

A. Manifestations

- Heart—pericarditis.
- Lungs—pleuritis.
- Renal disease.
- Skin lesions—erythematous rash in butterfly pattern on cheeks and across nose.

B. Lab Findings

- Antinuclear antibody (ANA) is initial test.
- Anti-dsDNA and anti-Sm are highly specific.
- Antiphospholipid antibodies.
- C3 and C4 complement levels will be low.
- Erythrocyte sedimentation rate (ESR) and C-reactive protein (CRP).

C. Hand Involvement

- Symmetric joint swelling.[28]
- Pain with motion.
- Morning stiffness.
- Raynaud's disease.
- Jaccoud's arthropathy—hypermobility of multiple joints due to ligamentous laxity.
- Joint deformities—absence of articular cartilage destruction and joint space narrowing seen in other forms of arthritis.
  - Volar plate laxity.
  - Tendon subluxation—extensor tendon subluxes ulnar to the metacarpal head.
  - Digital ulnar deviation and volar subluxation at MCP joint level.
  - Loss of active and then passive finger extension.
  - Thumb—often first place where hand deformity occurs:
    - MCP joint hyperextension or flexion—distal joint assumes opposite position.
    - Lateral subluxation of distal joint.
    - Subluxation or dislocation of CMC joint.

D. Wrist Involvement

- Scapholunate dissociation.
- Ulnar translocation of the carpus.
- Complete wrist dislocation.
- Carpal supination leading to prominence of the distal ulna:
  ○ Pain.
  ○ Reduced range of motion.
  ○ Extensor tendon ruptures from attrition.

E. Management

- Medical
  ○ NSAIDs.
  ○ Corticosteroids.
  ○ Antimalarial drugs—hydroxychloroquine and chloroquine.
- Splinting and hand therapy: Initial treatment of passively correctable deformities:
  ○ Wrists splints to maintain alignment.
  ○ Resting splints at night to properly align fingers at MCP joint level.
  ○ Silver Ring splint for swan neck deformities.
  ○ Soft-Core Foam™ splints for early boutonniere deformity.
- Surgical
  ○ Wrist surgeries[29]
    – Total wrist fusion for dislocation.
    – Wrist realignment with radiolunate or radiocarpal fusion for ulnar translocation of wrist.
    – Darrach's procedure with ECU stabilization to prevent dorsal migration.
  ○ Hand surgeries
    – Soft tissue realignment (deformity often recurs): Extensor tendon realignment or tenodesis.
    – Silicone arthroplasty for MCP deformity.[28]
    – Attachment of extensor tendon to proximal phalanx to prevent subluxation
    – Fusion for IP joint deformity.
    – Thumb surgeries: EPL rerouting—restores active MCP extension or MCP and CMC joint arthrodesis.

References

[1] Kaye BR, Kaye RL, Bobrove A. Rheumatoid nodules: review of the spectrum of associated conditions and proposal of a new classification, with a report of four seronegative cases. Am J Med. 1984; 76(2):279–292

[2] Malipeddi A, Reddy VR, Kallarackal G. Posterior interosseous nerve palsy: an unusual complication of rheumatoid arthritis: case report and review of the literature. Semin Arthritis Rheum. 2011; 40(6):576–579

[3] Backdahl M. The caput ulnae syndrome in rheumatoid arthritis: a study of the morphology, abnormal anatomy and clinical picture. Acta Rheumatol Scand Suppl. 1963; 5:1–75

[4] Mannerfelt L, Norman O. Attrition ruptures of flexor tendons in rheumatoid arthritis caused by bony spurs in the carpal tunnel: a clinical and radiological study. J Bone Joint Surg Br. 1969; 51(2):270–277

[5] Krause ML, Matteson EL. Perioperative management of the patient with rheumatoid arthritis. World J Orthop. 2014; 5(3):283–291

[6] Ouellette EA. The rheumatoid hand: orthotics as preventative. Semin Arthritis Rheum. 1991; 21(2):65–72

[7] Philips CA. Management of the patient with rheumatoid arthritis: the role of the hand therapist. Hand Clin. 1989; 5(2):291–309

[8] Nakagawa N, Yokoyama H, Matsuda S, Terashima Y, Kohyama K, Imura S. Short-term outcome of finger joint synovectomy in rheumatoid arthritis. Mod Rheumatol. 2011; 21(6):598–601

[9] Rozental TD. Reconstruction of the rheumatoid thumb. J Am Acad Orthop Surg. 2007; 15(2):118–125

[10] O'Sullivan MB, Singh H, Wolf JM. Tendon transfers in the rheumatoid hand for reconstruction. Hand Clin. 2016; 32(3):407–416

[11] Chung KC, Kowalski CP, Myra Kim H, Kazmers IS. Patient outcomes following Swanson silastic metacarpophalangeal joint arthroplasty in the rheumatoid hand: a systematic overview. J Rheumatol. 2000; 27(6):1395–1402

[12] Chalmers PN, Sherman SL, Raphael BS, Su EP. Rheumatoid synovectomy: does the surgical approach matter? Clin Orthop Relat Res. 2011; 469(7):2062–2071

[13] Grawe B, Heincelman C, Stern P. Functional results of the Darrach procedure: a long-term outcome study. J Hand Surg Am. 2012; 37(12):2475–80.e1, 2

[14] Lluch A. The Sauvé-Kapandji procedure: indications and tips for surgical success. Hand Clin. 2010; 26 (4):559–572

[15] Toma CD, Machacek P, Bitzan P, Assadian O, Trieb K, Wanivenhaus A. Fusion of the wrist in rheumatoid arthritis: a clinical and functional evaluation of two surgical techniques. J Bone Joint Surg Br. 2007; 89 (12):1620–1626

[16] Valdovinos ST, Landry GJ. Raynaud syndrome. Tech Vasc Interv Radiol. 2014; 17(4):241–246

[17] Williams AA, Carl HM, Lifchez SD. The scleroderma hand: manifestations of disease and approach to management. J Hand Surg Am. 2018; 43(6):550–557

[18] Thompson AE, Shea B, Welch V, Fenlon D, Pope JE. Calcium-channel blockers for Raynaud's phenomenon in systemic sclerosis. Arthritis Rheum. 2001; 44(8):1841–1847

[19] Roustit M, Blaise S, Allanore Y, Carpentier PH, Caglayan E, Cracowski JL. Phosphodiesterase-5 inhibitors for the treatment of secondary Raynaud's phenomenon: systematic review and meta-analysis of randomised trials. Ann Rheum Dis. 2013; 72(10):1696–1699

[20] Bogoch ER, Gross DK. Surgery of the hand in patients with systemic sclerosis: outcomes and considerations. J Rheumatol. 2005; 32(4):642–648

[21] Gilbart MK, Jolles BM, Lee P, Bogoch ER. Surgery of the hand in severe systemic sclerosis. J Hand Surg [Br]. 2004; 29(6):599–603

[22] Flatt AE. Digital artery sympathectomy. J Hand Surg Am. 1980; 5(6):550–556

[23] Uppal L, Dhaliwal K, Butler PE. A prospective study of the use of botulinum toxin injections in the treatment of Raynaud's syndrome associated with scleroderma. J Hand Surg Eur Vol. 2014; 39(8):876–880

[24] Bello RJ, Cooney CM, Melamed E, et al. The therapeutic efficacy of botulinum toxin in treating scleroderma-associated Raynaud's phenomenon: a randomized, double-blind, placebo-controlled clinical trial. Arthritis Rheumatol. 2017; 69(8):1661–1669

[25] Haddad A, Johnson SR, Somaily M, et al. Psoriatic arthritis mutilans: clinical and radiographic criteria. A systematic review. J Rheumatol. 2015; 42(8):1432–1438

[26] Day MS, Nam D, Goodman S, Su EP, Figgie M. Psoriatic arthritis. J Am Acad Orthop Surg. 2012; 20(1):28–37

[27] Gossec L, Smolen JS. Treatment of psoriatic arthritis: management recommendations. Clin Exp Rheumatol. 2015; 33(5) Suppl 93:S73–S77

[28] Fontaine C, Staumont-Sallé D, Hatron PY, Cotten A, Couturier C. The hand in systemic diseases other than rheumatoid arthritis. Chir Main. 2014; 33(3):155–173

[29] Nalebuff EA. Surgery of systemic lupus erythematosus arthritis of the hand. Hand Clin. 1996; 12(3):591–602

12 Tendinitis, Tendinosis, and Dupuytren's Contracture

Noah Raizman

Abstract

Tendinitis refers to acute inflammation due to acute damage or overuse. Tendinosis refers to chronic, often attritional damage due to overuse, abnormal anatomy, or degenerative conditions. There is significant overlap. "Tendinopathy" encompasses both. They may affect any flexor or extensor tendons, typically within a sheath or at inflection point, but may also affect tendon origin/insertions, in which case they are considered enthesopathies. Understanding the anatomy of the hand, wrist and elbow is key to diagnosis. History can elucidate mechanism and help isolate pathology in most cases and advanced imaging is rarely indicated. Management is often conservative at the outset, with surgical treatment indicated in recalcitrant cases. Dupuytren disease, a fibroproliferative genetic condition of incomplete penetrance, may lead to the evolution of cords and nodules in the hand and fingers. Treatment is typically reserved for cases leading to significant contracture and consists primarily of surgery, needle aponeurotomy or collagenase injection.

Keywords: Tendinitis, tendinosis, enthesopathy, tennis elbow, lateral epicondylitis, medial epicondylitis, golfer's elbow, dequervains, trigger finger, stenosing tenosynovitis, Dupuytren/Dupuytren's disease/contracture, intersection syndrome

I. Tendinitis and Tendinosis of Hand and Wrist

- *Tendinitis* refers to acute inflammation due to acute damage or overuse. *Tendinosis* refers to chronic, often attritional damage due to overuse, abnormal anatomy, or degenerative conditions. There is significant overlap. "*Tendinopathy*" encompasses both.
- They may affect any flexor or extensor tendons, typically within a sheath or at inflection point, but may also affect tendon origin/insertions, in which case they are considered *enthesopathies*.
- Avoid giving diagnosis of "tendinitis" to patients with nonspecific overuse pain. Nonspecific or specific overuse pain that is seemingly related to occupation may benefit from a formal ergonomic assessment versus self-directed activity modification.
- History can elucidate mechanism and help isolate pathology in most cases. Physical examination is usually confirmatory. Special diagnostic tests such as MRI and ultrasound are necessary only in specific cases and should not be ordered without clear reason.
- Understanding location of the six extensor compartments at the wrist (▶ Fig. 12.1) and flexor and extensor tendon anatomy is key to diagnosis.

A. Wrist Flexor/Extensor Tendinitis

- Flexor carpi radialis (FCR)
  - Tender over FCR, typically close to distal pole of scaphoid.

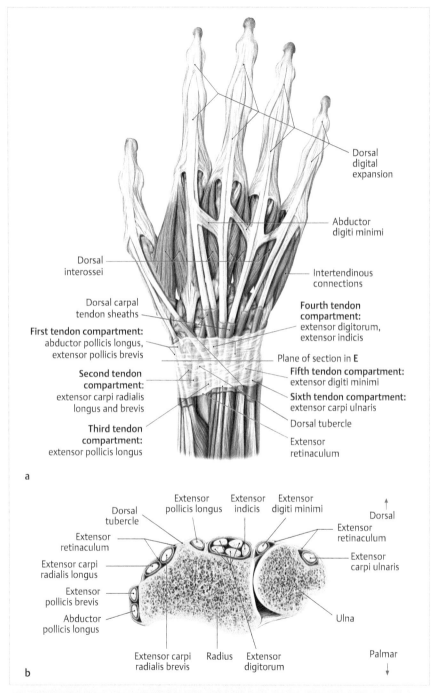

Fig. 12.1 (a) Extensor retinaculum and dorsal carpal tendon sheaths. (b) Schematic cross-section through the forearm at the level of the distal radioulnar joint. Source: Schünke M, Schulte E, Schumacher U et al., ed. THIEME Atlas of Anatomy, Volume 1: General Anatomy and Musculoskeletal System. 2nd ed. Thieme; 2014. Illustration by Karl Wesker/Markus Voll.

- ○ Pain with resisted wrist flexion.
- ○ Treated with splinting, occupational therapy (OT), and nonsteroidal anti-inflammatory drugs (NSAIDs).
- ○ Corticosteroid injection (CSI) sometimes useful, surgery rarely indicated.
- Flexor carpi ulnaris (FCU)
  - ○ Typically just proximal to pisiform.
  - ○ Treated similarly to FCR.
  - ○ MRI may be indicated to differentiate from pisotriquetral arthritis.
- Extensor carpi radialis longus (ECRL) and extensor carpi radialis brevis (ECRB)
  - ○ Typically manifests as intersection syndrome proximally (see below).
  - ○ May be associated with carpal boss—overgrowth/enthesopathy involving 2nd/3rd carpometacarpal (CMC) joint at the level of insertion of the wrist extensors.
    - Conservative treatment, with splinting, activity modification, rarely CSI, and surgical intervention with craterization of boss with or without CMC fusion and tendon repair is rarely needed.

B. Stenosing Tenosynovitis—"Trigger Finger"

- Thickening of flexor tendon at the level of A1 pulley with eventual formation of nodule of inflammatory tissue at the level of Camper's chiasm (▶ Fig. 12.2).
- Tenderness with or without palpable nodule at A1 pulley.

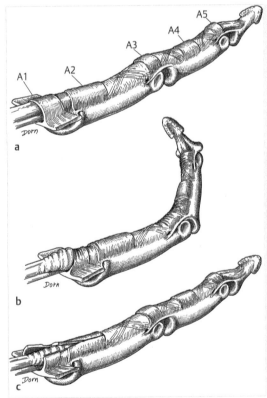

Fig. 12.2 **(a)** A nodule within the flexor tendons in the tendon sheath of a finger glides freely back and forth so long as the nodule is within the sheath. **(b)** With finger flexion, the tendon with the nodule moves proximally out of the sheath into the open palm. As the finger is extended, it "wads up" against the clifflike entrance of the tight sheath, which increases its size. **(c)** Surgical treatment of finger flexor tenosynovitis is to split longitudinally the A1 pulley, thus converting the entrance of the sheath into a funnel configuration into which even the enlarged tendon enters readily. Alternatively, for those with unusually skillful demands of their hands, such as professional musicians, only a few millimeters of the sheath's entrance is incised, and the diameter of the flexor digitorum superficialis (FDS) tendon is reduced by excision of a long elliptical wedge from its center. The two sides fall together without sutures. Source: Beasley R, ed. Beasley's Surgery of the Hand. Thieme; 2003.

- May be associated with retinacular cyst.
- Early—just pain, progresses to "locking".
- Grading
  - Pain, no clicking.
  - Pain, clicking, easily reducible.
  - Must be reduced manually.
  - Locked, irreducible.
- Initial treatment
  - CSI 90 + % effective, approximately 70% long-term efficacy
    - Less effective in diabetes mellitus (DM).
    - May try up to three CSI (decreased efficacy with repeated injection).
  - Nighttime extension splinting and physical therapy (PT)/OT may be effective in reducing symptoms.
- Surgical treatment
  - Release of A1 pulley—can be performed under local anesthesia.
  - Recurrence rate very low (< 5%) after surgery.
  - Failed surgery may require re-release with release of A0 and proximal A2 pulleys versus excision of one slip of flexor digitorum superficialis (FDS).

C. De Quervain's Tenosynovitis

- Tendinitis of first dorsal compartment (abductor pollicis longus [APL] and extensor pollicis brevis [EPB]) (▶ Fig. 12.3).
- Very common in general population, with specific history of repetitive lifting or ulnar deviation/flexion; extremely common in post-partum mothers ("Mommy Wrist").
- Physical examination
  - Tenderness of 1st dorsal compartment with or without swelling.
  - Finkelstein's test—traction and flexion/palmar abduction of thumb reproduces symptoms.

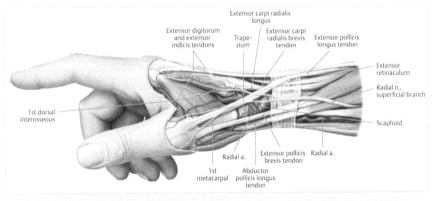

Fig. 12.3 Right hand, radial view. The three-sided "anatomic snuffbox" (*shaded light yellow*) is bounded by the tendons of insertion of the abductor pollicis longus and the extensor pollicis brevis and extensor pollicis longus. Source: Gilroy A, Voll M, Wesker K, ed. Anatomy: An Essential Textbook. 2nd ed. Thieme; 2017. Illustration by Karl Wesker/Markus Voll.

- Initial treatment
  - CSI highly effective (90 + %).
  - Separate subsheath between APL and EPB may be the cause of failure, when present.
  - Thumb spica splinting and OT may be of moderate benefit.
- Surgical treatment
  - Open release:
    - Avoid damage or traction to radial sensory nerve.
    - Must release both APL and EPB—look for subsheath.

D. Intersection Syndrome

- Irritation of extensor tendons (notably the radial wrist extensors) underneath brachioradialis.
- Characterized by swelling/crepitus and tenderness 5 to 8 cm proximal to wrist, dorsoradially.
- CSI usually curative.

E. Extensor (Extensor Pollicis Longus [EPL]/Extensor Digitorum Communis [EDC]/ Extensor Digitorum Minimi [EDM]) Tendinitis

- Tenderness and swelling over extensor compartments.
- May be overuse/exertion related.
- May respond to rest/splinting and hand therapy with or without NSAIDs.

F. Extensor Carpi Ulnaris (ECU) Tendinitis/Instability

- ECU subsheath prevents subluxation with wrist ulnar deviated and supinated; damage to subsheath may cause either pain, subluxation, or instability.
- Common in golfers, racket sport players, and baseball players.
- Clearly acute dislocation/subluxation or pain without instability may respond to trial of Munster splint immobilization and rest with or without CSI. Consider taping of ECU in athletes for return to sport.
- Chronic injuries or those failing initial conservative management may require surgical stabilization.
  - Sheath may be reconstructed with suture anchors (Graham) or with extensor retinaculum. Deepening of groove is commonly performed but unlikely to be necessary for stability.

II. Tendinopathy of the Elbow

A. Lateral Epicondylitis "Tennis Elbow"

- Overload injury to origin of ECRB.
- Most common cause of elbow pain; affects 1 to 3% of adults annually, peaking in 40s to 50s.
- Best referred to as "lateral elbow tendinopathy" as it is minimally inflammatory and located just distal to epicondyle.

- Pathology is angiofibroblastic hyperplasia with minimal inflammation and disorganized collagen.
- Diagnosis: Characteristic tenderness over ECRB origin:
  - Pain with resisted wrist extension.
  - No indication for MRI.
- Treatment is most often conservative, as the condition is usually self-limited and resolves spontaneously in 80 to 90% of patients.
  - Activity modification.
  - Wrist brace (unloads extensors) versus counterforce brace ("tennis elbow strap")—equivalent efficacy in literature.
  - PT similarly effective to expectant management, no clear difference between eccentric or concentric strengthening.
  - CSI, while effective in the short term, has been shown in multiple studies to either have no effect on ultimate disease course, or else to lead to worse functional outcomes at 12 months.
  - Autologous blood and platelet-rich plasma (PRP) injections have seemingly shown to be effective in small studies, only when compared to CSI. When compared to placebo, no randomized clinical trial (RCT) has shown efficacy.
  - Multiple additional modalities (shockwave, acupuncture, phonophoresis, prolotherapy, dry needling, etc.) have not been shown conclusively to affect outcome.
- Surgical treatment
  - Indicated after at least 6 to 12 months of conservative treatment.
  - Percutaneous tenotomy (with or without ultrasound guidance), arthroscopic debridement, and open surgical debridement of ECRB with or without repair all show similar long-term outcomes (75–85% success rates overall) in few comparison studies. Iatrogenic lateral ulnar collateral ligament injury is potential complication.

B. Medial Epicondylitis

- Similar to lateral elbow tendinopathy in terms of pathophysiology.
- Localized to flexor/pronator origin.
- Treatment paradigm identical to lateral epicondylitis.

C. Biceps/Triceps Tendinosis

- Typically degenerative and chronic or acute-on-chronic in nature.
- Triceps tendinitis
  - Conservative treatment usually effective.
  - Avoid CSI for fear of tendon rupture.
- Biceps tendinitis
  - MRI may show partial tearing of biceps.
  - Treatment is conservative for 3 to 4 months.
  - If pain continues, can consider takedown and reinsertion of biceps tendon with good reported outcomes.

III. Dupuytren's Contracture

- Benign proliferative disorder characterized by formation of abnormal thickenings of palmar and digital aponeurotic system (cords and nodules) (▶ Fig. 12.4).

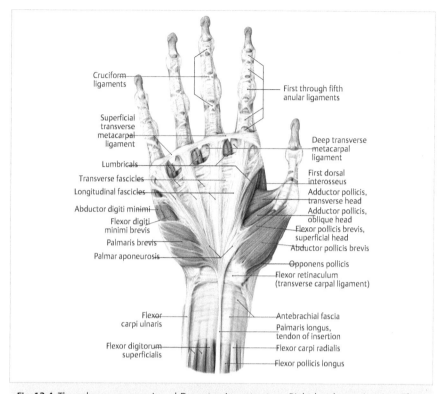

Cruciform ligaments

Superficial transverse metacarpal ligament

Lumbricals

Transverse fascicles

Longitudinal fascicles

Abductor digiti minimi

Flexor digiti minimi brevis

Palmaris brevis

Palmar aponeurosis

Flexor carpi ulnaris

Flexor digitorum superficialis

First through fifth anular ligaments

Deep transverse metacarpal ligament

First dorsal interosseus

Adductor pollicis, transverse head

Adductor pollicis, oblique head

Flexor pollicis brevis, superficial head

Abductor pollicis brevis

Opponens pollicis

Flexor retinaculum (transverse carpal ligament)

Antebrachial fascia

Palmaris longus, tendon of insertion

Flexor carpi radialis

Flexor pollicis longus

Fig. 12.4 The palmar aponeurosis and Dupuytren's contracture. Right hand, anterior view. The muscular fascia of the palm is thickened by firm connective tissue to form the palmar aponeurosis, which separates the palm from the subcutaneous fat to protect the soft tissues. Source: Schünke M, Schulte E, Schumacher U et al., ed. THIEME Atlas of Anatomy, Volume 1: General Anatomy and Musculoskeletal System. 2nd ed. Thieme; 2014.

- Genetics: Autosomal dominant with variable penetrance, multiple potential implicated genes, associated with Northern European descent.
- Named for Guillaume Dupuytren, chief surgeon of the Hotel de Dieu in Paris during the Napoleonic wars who described surgical treatment in 1831; however, Sir Astley Cooper described percutaneous aponeurotomy for the condition 10 years earlier.
- Pathophysiology: Myofibroblasts predominance, associated with Type III collagen (40%), multiple factors implicated, namely, IL-1, PDGF, FGF, TGF-β, as well as downregulation of matrix metalloproteinases (MMPs).
- Risk factors include HIV, smoking, alcoholism, DM, anti-seizure medications, and trauma (acute or repetitive).
- Ectopic disease: Garrod's disease (knuckle pads), Ledderhose's disease (plantar fascia), and Peyronie's disease (Dartos' fascia of the penis).
- Diagnosis: Presence of stereotypical stigmata—nodules, cords with or without contracture, and skin pitting.
- Characteristic cords (▶ Fig. 12.5).
  ○ Pretendinous
    – Palmar, overlying tendons, typically straight.

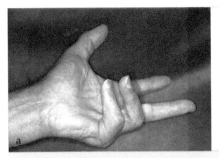
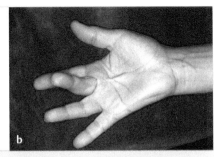

Fig. 12.5 (a) Typical established Dupuytren's disease. It can involve any part of the hand, but usually the medial side (middle, ring, and small fingers) is most involved. **(b)** Typical Dupuytren's contractures. Source: Beasley R, ed. Beasley's Surgery of the Hand. Thieme; 2003.

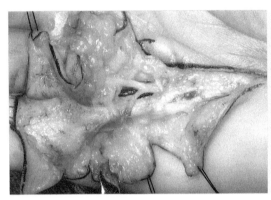

Fig. 12.6 At the base of the proximal phalanges any anatomic arrangement can be encountered. Illustrated is a digital nerve crossing over and spiraling around a diseased pretendinous fascial band. Dissection in this area should be just deep to the skin until there has been positive identification of the neurovascular bundles. Source: Beasley R, ed. Beasley's Surgery of the Hand. Thieme; 2003.

  – Continuous with central cord, which causes MCP contracture.
- ○ Natatory cord—cause webspace contracture.
- ○ Spiral cord—causes proximal interphalangeal (PIP) contracture:
  – Comprises thickened/abnormal pretendinous band, spiral band, Grayson's ligament, and lateral digital sheet.
  – Spirals underneath neurovascular (NV) bundle, displacing it centrally/volarly—surgical risk (▶ Fig. 12.6).
- ○ Retrovascular cord
  – Runs from P1 to P3, dorsal to NV bundle.
  – Associated with distal interphalangeal (DIP) contracture.
- ○ Skin pitting: Fibrosis of Grapow's fibers.
- ○ Nodules: Focal thickening.

A. Treatment

- • Conservative therapy
  - ○ Prophylactic splinting and range of motion (ROM) exercises of limited benefit.
  - ○ Interventional treatment usually indicated when patient fails the "table top test"—(i.e., has enough contracture that palm cannot be placed flat on table).

- Clostridium histolyticum collagenase
  - Enzyme derived from bacteria, injected into cords, followed by manipulation.
  - Preferable to Type I and Type III collagen (spares Type IV).
  - Major potential complication is flexor tendon rupture—0.2% (most likely at small finger PIP); other complications include skin tearing, swelling/ecchymosis, and lymphadenopathy.
  - Approximately 35% recurrence at 3 years follow-up.
- Percutaneous needle aponeurotomy
  - Office-based.
  - Local anesthesia to skin, superficially.
  - 22 or 25gauge needle.
  - May be repeated, but has relatively high recurrence rate.
  - Ideal for isolated pretendinous cords.
- Surgical fasciectomy
  - Limited fasciectomy:
    - Removal of most, but not all, Dupuytren's tissue, maintaining skin.
    - Most commonly performed surgical procedure.
    - Limited: Multiple small incisions versus regional—Bruner versus V-Y versus Z-plasty.
    - 15 to 43% recurrence at 3 years.
  - McCash open palm
    - Limited fasciectomy, leaving palmar incisions open to heal by secondary intention.
    - Rarely performed.
  - Radical fasciectomy
    - Removal of all Dupuytren's tissue and entire aponeurotic system with wide exposure—highly morbid, rarely performed.
  - Dermatofasciectomy
    - Removal of both Dupuytren's tissue and overlying skin.
    - Full-thickness skin graft (FTSG).
    - Can be performed in limited fashion.
    - Lower rates of recurrence compared to limited fasciectomy.
    - Removing skin and grafting often paired with limited fasciectomy in the setting of prior surgery, chronic PIP contracture, etc.

B. Adjunctive Treatment

- Radiation therapy
  - Some European studies suggest slowing of progression in mild disease; not commonly practiced in the US.
- Skeletal traction
  - Very effective adjunct for ligamentous/capsular PIP contractures.
  - Typically applied for 6 to 10 weeks prior to fasciectomy.

C. Outcomes and Expectations

- Dupuytren's contracture is a disease that hand surgeons treat but do not cure.
- Even the best surgical procedures show significant recurrence rates.

- In Dupuytren's diathesis (those with early onset in 20s to 30s, often bilateral and multiple fingers involved, often associated with Ledderhose's or Peyronie's disease or Garrod's pads), no treatment is likely to provide more than temporary improvement.
- Progression is difficult, if not impossible, to predict.
- Patients need to understand the chronic and often unrelenting nature of the disease.

13 Infection

R. Timothy Kreulen and Dawn LaPorte

Keywords: Hand infection, sepsis, incision and drainage

Abstract

Infections in the hand are a common and diverse group of conditions. The physician's evaluation begins with an overall assessment of the patient, including past medical history, allergies, occupation, and activities. Assessment continues with the history, physical examination, imaging, and laboratory testing to make a diagnosis. Once a diagnosis has been made, treatment should be initiated. Timing of treatment often impacts prognosis and patient outcomes. It is imperative that the treating physician understand the common hand infection conditions so that patients can receive timely and proper treatment.

Keywords: Hand infection, sepsis, incision and drainage

I. Patient Evaluation

- Stabilize patient
  - First priority is treating sepsis if present with broad spectrum antibiotics and intravenous (IV) fluid administration.
- History
  - Time of onset.
  - Mechanism.
  - Occupation, handedness, social situation, and activity level.
  - Medical evaluation of comorbidities, allergies (especially to antibiotics), anticipate risks with anesthesia or surgery.
- Physical examination
  - Location of symptoms on flexor versus extensor surfaces.
  - Erythema, swelling, gross purulence, crepitus, and fluid collections.
  - Pain with palpation or passive movement of fingers/wrist.
- Preoperative tests
  - Blood cultures if worried about systemic infection, ideally before antibiotics.
  - Complete blood count (CBC), basic metabolic panel (BMP), prothrombin time and international normalized ratio (PT/INR), partial thromboplastin time (PTT), type and screen.
  - Electrocardiogram (EKG) and chest X-ray based upon medical history.

II. Important Infections

A. Necrotizing Fasciitis

- Background
  - Life and limb threatening surgical emergency.
  - Bacterial spread along fascial planes.

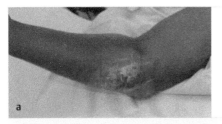 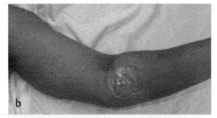

Fig. 13.1 (a, b) Upper extremity with erythema, skin sloughing, and bullae, consistent with necrotizing fasciitis.

- Presentation
  - Pain.
  - Bullae, cutaneous hemorrhage, skin sloughing, and crepitus (▶ Fig. 13.1).
  - Most commonly caused by polymicrobial infection; most common isolated organism is Group A strep.
- Testing
  - Imaging not required for diagnosis but may show gas in tissue planes.
  - Labs consistent with inflammatory/infectious process: LRINEC scoring (score ≥6 predictive of necrotizing fasciitis).
    - C-reactive protein (CRP) ≥15 = 4 points.
    - WBC <15 = 0 points; 15–25 = 1 point; >25 = 2 points.
    - Hemoglobin >13.5 = 0 points; 11–13.5 = 1 point; <11 = 2 points.
    - Sodium ≥135 = 2 points.
    - Creatinine >1.6 = 2 points.
    - Glucose ≥180 = 2 points.
- Treatment
  - Surgical emergency—incision and drainage (remove all necrotic tissue) versus amputation with obtaining intraoperative cultures.
    - Timing to operating room (OR) most important factor in survival.
    - Risk factors for poor outcome are delay in time to OR, age >50 years, and diabetes.
    - Classically see "dishwater" fluid from liquefied fat intraoperatively.
  - Broad spectrum IV antibiotics
    - Empiric antibiotics: Penicillin G, clindamycin, metronidazole, and aminoglycoside.
    - Strep or clostridium: Penicillin G.
    - Polymicrobial: Imipenem, doripenem, or meropenem.
    - Methicillin-resistant Staphylococcus aureus (MRSA): Vancomycin or daptomycin.

B. Septic Arthritis

- Background
  - Infection within a joint.
  - Cartilage can be destroyed secondary to release of bacterial toxins and proteolytic enzymes.
  - Most common organism is *Staphylococcus aureus*, but consider *Neisseria gonorrhoeae* in those with risk factors.

- Presentation
  - Swollen, painful joint with decreased range of motion; pain with active and passive range of motion; pain with axial loading of joint.
- Testing
  - Joint aspiration.
    - WBC >50,000, polymorphonuclear leukocytes >75%, glucose level 40 mg < fasting glucose.
- Treatment
  - Incision and drainage in OR with cultures.
  - Intravenous antibiotics.

C. Osteomyelitis

- Background
  - Infection of bone.
  - Risk factors include recent surgery, trauma, IV drug use immunocompromised state, poor blood supply, and neuropathy.
  - Most common organisms are *S. aureus* and *Streptococcus.*
  - Sequestrum is an area of dead bone near an infected nidus.
  - Involucrum is new bone forming around area of necrosis.
- Presentation
  - History of fever, although fever is usually only seen in acute cases.
  - Erythema, tenderness, and sinus tracts can all be seen on examination.
- Testing
  - Radiographs obtained first can show lucencies/sclerosis and periosteal reaction.
  - MRI with contrast best test to assess for extent of infection and assist in surgical planning (▸ Fig. 13.2).
  - CBC, erythrocyte sedimentation rate (ESR), CRP, and blood cultures should be obtained.
- Treatment
  - Nonoperative
    - Only when operative intervention is not possible.

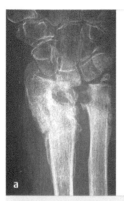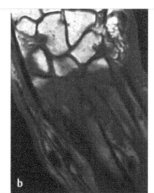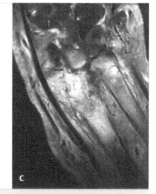

Fig. 13.2 (a) X-ray demonstrating periosteal reaction and diffuse sclerosis. (b) T1- and (c) T2- weighted MRI showing bone and soft tissue inflammation, consistent with osteomyelitis.

- Operative
  - Irrigation and debridement of all devitalized tissue; advanced cases may require amputation.
  - Obtain intraoperative or preoperative cultures to narrow antibiotics.
- Antibiotics
  - Tailor based on bone cultures.

D. Flexor Tenosynovitis

- Background
  - Infection in the flexor tendon sheath.
  - Mechanism: Typically direct inoculation of bacteria from puncture, bite, or spread from nearby abscess.
  - Missed diagnosis can lead to stiffness, tendon or pulley rupture, spread of the infection.
  - Most common organism is *S. aureus*.
- Presentation
  - Kanavel signs (▶ Fig. 13.3):
    - Flexed position.
    - Flexor sheath tenderness.
    - Fusiform swelling.
    - Pain with passive extension.
  - Pain and swelling on flexor side.
- Testing
  - X-rays to look for foreign body and air.
  - Labs: CBC, ESR, CRP, and blood cultures.
- Treatment
  - Nonoperative
    - If examination is equivocal, can admit to hospital for 24-hour trial of IV antibiotics, soft tissue rest/immobilization.
    - If symptoms fail to improve, must go to the OR.
    - It is rare to manage flexor tenosynovitis nonoperatively.
  - Operative
    - Incision and drainage flexor sheath in OR.
    - Obtain cultures.
    - Treat postoperatively with culture-specific antibiotic regimen.

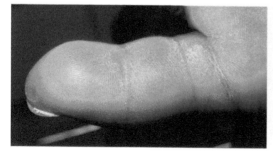

Fig. 13.3 Finger held in flexed position with fusiform swelling, consistent with flexor tenosynovitis.

E. Felon

- Background
  - Infection of finger pulp.
  - Fingertip pulp is separated into many closed sacs of connective tissue by fibrous vertical septations.
  - Most common organism is *S. aureus.*
- Presentation
  - Pain and swelling on volar fingertip.
  - Pointing abscess.
  - May drain actively.
- Testing
  - Consider X-ray to rule out foreign body or if patient has history of trauma.
  - Labs typically not indicated.
- Treatment
  - Bedside incision and drainage:
    - Perform digital block.
    - Make incision over mid-lateral or directly over volar aspect of finger.
    - Stay distal to distal interphalangeal (DIP) joint.
    - Break up septa to decompress infection.
    - Leave open and pack wound.
  - Culture if possible.
  - IV versus oral culture-specific antibiotics.

F. Paronychia/Eponychia

- Background
  - Nail fold infections:
    - Infection at base of nail fold is an eponychia.
    - Infection on radial/ulnar nail fold is a paronychia.
  - Most common hand infection.
  - Most common bacteria is *S. aureus.*
  - Acute versus chronic:
    - Acute—trauma from nail biting, thumb sucking, etc.
    - Chronic—occupations with chronic exposure to chemicals/bacteria like dishwashers, especially in those with medical comorbidities.
- Presentation
  - Pain, swelling, and erythema at nail fold.
  - Tenderness and potential fluctuance on examination.
- Testing
  - Imaging typically not indicated unless there is concern for foreign body or osteomyelitis.
  - Laboratory testing typically not indicated.
- Treatment
  - Acute infection
    - Nonoperative: Warm soapy soaks, oral antibiotics, and avoidance of inciting event.
    - Operative: Bedside incision and drainage with partial or total nail bed removal (▶ Fig. 13.4).

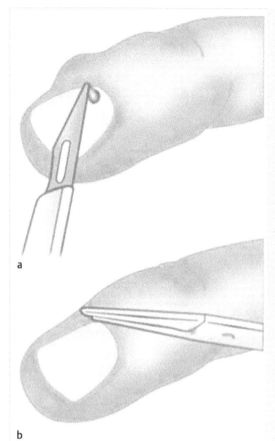

Fig. 13.4 Paronychia **(a)** before and **(b)** after proper incision and drainage with a scalpel.

a

b

- ○ Chronic infection
  - – Nonoperative: Warm soapy soaks, avoidance of inciting event, and topical antifungal like miconazole.
  - – Operative: Marsupialization, meaning incise dorsal eponychium down to germinal matrix.

G. Deep Infections

- Background
  - ○ Infection in deep spaces.
  - ○ Common locations:
    - – Thenar space: Radial muscle group.
    - – Hypothenar space: Ulnar muscle group.
    - – Midpalmar space: Space between flexor tendons and metacarpals.
    - – Parona's space: Space between flexor tendons and pronator quadratus.
    - – Collar button abscess: Webspace between fingers (▶ Fig. 13.5).

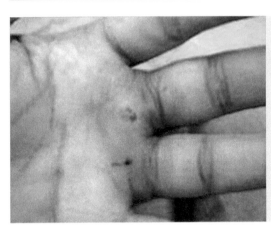

Fig. 13.5 Purulent drainage, erythema, and swelling in the webspace consistent with a collar button abscess.

- Presentation
  - Pain and swelling.
  - Potential history of trauma.
  - Pain with palpation over infected area or with flexion of tendons running through infected space.
- Testing
  - X-rays can help rule out a foreign body and reassure that there is no free air.
  - Ultrasound, MRI with contrast, or CT with contrast may be indicated to define extent of infection.
  - Consider CBC, ESR, CRP, and blood cultures.
- Treatment
  - Incision and drainage, typically in OR.
  - IV antibiotics.

H. Herpetic Whitlow

- Background
  - Infection with herpes simplex virus (HSV-1 or HSV-2).
  - Self-limited.
  - Common in dental workers and toddlers.
- Presentation
  - Vesicular lesions that initially drain and then mature into ulcers (▶ Fig. 13.6).
  - Lymphadenitis.
- Testing
  - Imaging and labs typically not indicated.
  - Consider Tzanck smear of vesicle fluid.
- Treatment
  - Acyclovir.
  - NOT incision and drainage.

I. Sporotrichosis

- Background

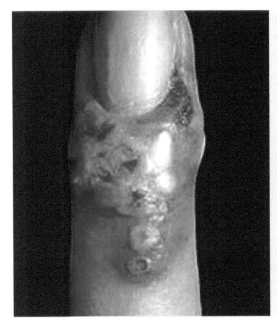

Fig. 13.6 Erythematous vesicles covering finger consistent with herpetic whitlow.

- Infection with fungus *Sporothrix schenckii*, which is commonly found in rose thorns.
- Commonly seen in gardeners.
- Presentation
  - Erythematous nodule(s).
  - Can be associated with erythematous rashes in later cases.
- Testing
  - Imaging typically not indicated.
  - Labs typically not indicated.
- Treatment
  - Oral itraconazole for 3 to 6 months.
  - Formerly was treated with potassium iodide, which has fallen out of favor due to side effects.

J. Bite Wounds

- Background
  - Determine if bite is from human or animal.
  - If human, "fight bites" are commonly found:
    - Located on dorsum of hand.
    - Bacteria may inoculate joint capsule.
  - If animal, dog bites are most common followed by cat bites.
- Presentation
  - History of bite/hand striking human or animal in mouth:
    - *Eikenella corrodens* seen with human bites.
    - *Pasteurella multocida* seen with dog bites.
  - Examination shows puncture wounds versus lacerations (▶ Fig. 13.7).
  - Important to note if wounds violate joint.

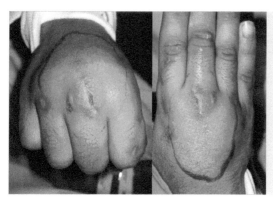

Fig. 13.7 Small, linear defects in hand at metacarpophalangeal (MCP) joint with surrounding erythema from a fight bite.

  ○ Pain, swelling, erythema, and purulence can all be seen.
- Testing
  ○ X-rays to make sure no tooth or other foreign object is retained.
  ○ Consider CBC, ESR, CRP, and culture if possible.
- Treatment
  ○ Tetanus and rabies prophylaxis if not up-to-date.
  ○ Antibiotics (IV TMP-SMX then oral amoxicillin-clavulanic acid).
  ○ Irrigation and debridement at bedside or in OR.
  ○ Consider immobilization for soft tissue rest.
  ○ Irrigation and debridement in OR for progressive infection after bedside treatment, foreign body, crush injuries, deep infections, and infections in the joint.

K. High-Pressure Injection Injuries

- Background
  ○ Commonly seen with laborers using paint gun with organic solvent.
  ○ Nondominant index finger most commonly injured.
  ○ High risk for amputation despite often benign appearing external injuries due to extensive soft tissue damage.
- Presentation
  ○ History of injection.
  ○ Entry wound can be benign looking, masking underlying soft tissue damage.
- Testing
  ○ X-rays to rule out foreign body (▶ Fig. 13.8).
  ○ Laboratory values usually not indicated.
- Treatment
  ○ Tetanus prophylaxis and antibiotics for all patients.
  ○ Consider nonoperative monitoring for injections of water or air.
  ○ Urgent operative irrigation and debridement for organic compounds (most cases).
  ○ Low threshold for fasciotomies due to risk of compartment syndrome.

L. Mycobacterial Infections

- Background
  ○ Nontuberculous mycobacterial infections.

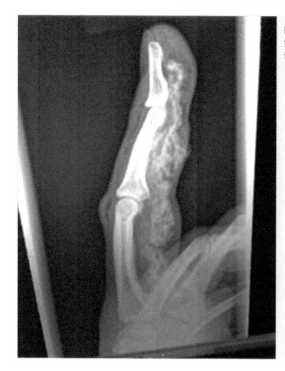

Fig. 13.8 Radiopaque material throughout flexor side of finger from high-pressure paint injury.

- ○ Most common in people with exposure to seawater and the immunocompromised.
- ○ Common organisms are *Mycobacterium marinum* (most common), *Mycobacterium kansasii*, *Mycobacterium terrae*, and *Mycobacterium aviumintracellularae.*
- Presentation
  - ○ Painful rash.
  - ○ May have lymphadenopathy.
- Testing
  - ○ Culture lesion on Lowenstein-Jensen agar.
- Treatment
  - ○ Nonoperative for those diagnosed early:
    - Antibiotics with trimethoprim-sulfamethoxazole, clarithromycin, azithromycin, ethambutol, and tetracycline.
    - Add rifampin for osteomyelitis.
  - ○ Operative for those diagnosed later:
    - Incision and drainage in OR with 3 to 6 months course of antibiotics.

M. Aeromonas Hydrophila from Leeches

- Background
  - ○ *Aeromonas hydrophila* lives symbiotically in the gut of many leeches.
  - ○ Bacteria can be spread to patient if leech therapy is utilized.
- Presentation
  - ○ Indications for leech therapy include treating venous congestion and debriding necrotic tissue.

- Diagnosis
  - No testing, but must consider prophylaxis whenever leeches are used.
- Treatment
  - Ciprofloxacin therapy used with leeches.
  - If there is a contraindication to ciprofloxacin, use trimethoprim-sulfamethoxazole.

Suggested Readings

Goldstein EJ. Bite wounds and infection. Clin Infect Dis 1992;14(3):633–638

Kennedy CD, Huang JI, Hanel DP. In brief: Kanavel's signs and pyogenic flexor tenosynovitis. Clin Orthop Relat Res. 2016; 474(1):280–284

Koshy JC, Bell B. Hand infections. J Hand Surg Am. 2019; 44(1):46–54

14 Flexor Tendon Injury, Repair, and Reconstruction

Nicole Schroeder

Abstract

Flexor tendon lacerations are disabling injuries that require surgeons to have an in-depth comprehension of anatomy, surgical techniques, and dedicated rehabilitation protocols in order to optimize functional outcome. While basic principles have remained constant, certain elements in management have evolved over the past three decades and will be discussed. Clinical outcomes of flexor tendon repair have significantly improved due to advances in suturing techniques and postoperative rehabilitation.

In this chapter, we will review the anatomy, basic principles and repair techniques for flexor tendon injuries, as well as select rehabilitation protocols. As primary repair is not an option in delayed presentation of flexor tendon injuries, we will also discuss potential reconstruction options. Despite all of this, successful outcomes are not always a guarantee as patient compliance with rehabilitation is critical.

Keywords: Flexor tendon anatomy, flexor tendon repair, flexor tendon rehabilitation, zone II, reconstruction

I. Anatomy

A. Flexor Tendon

- The flexor digitorum superficialis (FDS) is innervated in the forearm by the median nerve. The flexor digitorum profundus (FDP) lies deep to FDS and is innervated by the ulnar nerve (small and ring fingers) and the median nerve (index and long fingers).
- FDP has a common muscle belly, but index finger may arise independently. At the carpal tunnel, the FDS to index and small fingers lie beneath the ring and long fingers.
- Flexor tendons are divided into five zones (▶ Fig. 14.1).

B. Pulleys

- At the metacarpal neck, FDS and FDP enter a synovial sheath (A1 pulley). Here, the FDS splits (decussation) to allow FDP to become superficial. FDS slips then rejoin at Camper's chiasm (over proximal phalanx) and split again to insert on the middle phalanx.
- Pulley system (▶ Fig. 14.2): Five annular (A) and three cruciate (C) pulleys:
  - A1, 3, and 5 originate from the volar plates of the joints, while A2 and A4 arise from the volar bone of the proximal and middle phalanx, respectively.
  - C1, C2, and C3 lie between the A pulleys.

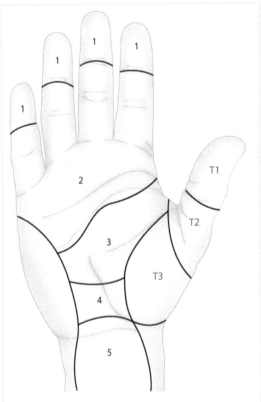

Fig. 14.1 Zones of flexor tendon injuries. Zone 1, distal to FDS insertion; Zone 2, proximal aspect of A1 pulley to FDS insertion; Zone 3, end of carpal tunnel to start of A1; Zone 4, carpal tunnel; Zone 5, forearm to carpal tunnel; T1, T2, T3: thumb zones.

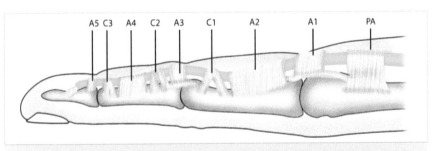

Fig. 14.2 Flexor pulley system. The pulley system is composed of both annular ligaments (A) and cruciate ligaments (C) and runs from A1 to A5. The A1 pulley begins over the metacarpal head, and the A5 pulley ends over the DIP joint.

C. Thumb

- Flexor pollicis longus (FPL) is innervated by the anterior interosseous nerve. The thumb pulley system consists of the A1, oblique (AO), and A2 pulleys. A1 and A2 originate off the volar plate of the metacarpophalangeal (MCP) and interphalangeal (IP) joints, whereas the A0 runs obliquely over proximal phalanx and is critical to FPL function. The oblique pulley is the most important for prevention of FPL bowstringing.

II. Tendon Biology

A. Nutrition (Two Sources)

- Synovial diffusion (imbibition).
- Direct blood supply: Vincula (short and long), intrinsic longitudinal vessels, FDP tendon insertion into distal phalanx, and proximal synovial fold.
- Each tendon has hypovascular zones located between the two vincula.

B. Tendon Histology

- Tendons consist of a cellular and acellular matrix of collagen (primarily Type I) and elastin, embedded within a proteoglycan–water matrix.
- Cross-linking of collagen molecules and the parallel alignment of the fibers make tendons ideal for tension bearing.

C. Tendon Healing

- Both intrinsic and extrinsic healing occur; extrinsic healing leads to adhesions, so goal is intrinsic healing.
- Three phases:
  - *Inflammatory* (day 1 to day 5): Inflammatory cells migrate into the repair site, leaving hematoma and granulation tissue. The strength of the repair is dependent on the suture. Highest risk for tendon rupture during this time.
  - *Proliferative* (day 5 to day 21): Fibroblasts migrate and collagen synthesis occurs—mainly type III collagen.
  - *Remodeling* (3 weeks to 6 months): Collagen organization and cross-linking occurs—mainly type I collagen. Repair gains tensile strength.

III. Patient Evaluation

A. Clinical Examination

- Look at finger cascade to see resting flexor tone (▶ Fig. 14.3).
- Check sensation distal to injury (radial and ulnar sides) and finger perfusion (doppler or pulse oximeter).
- Digital block *after* sensory examination can help to better assess motor examination.
  - Check FDS and FDP functions independently.
  - Assess for partial versus complete tendon laceration (visual inspection) and document percentage of laceration (if partial).

IV. Principles of Repair

- Fundamentals (Strickland): Easy placement of sutures in the tendon, secure suture knots, smooth juncture of the tendon ends, minimal gapping at the repair site,

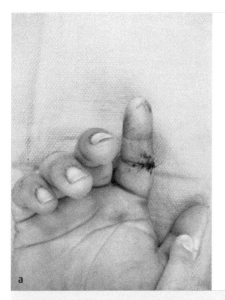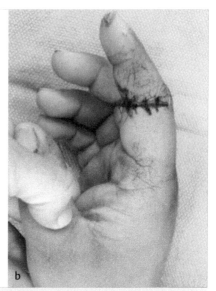

Fig. 14.3 (a, b) Resting posture showing asymmetry due to flexor tendon laceration in the index finger.

minimal interference with tendon vascularity, and sufficient strength throughout healing to permit application of early motion stress to the tendon.
- A repair is biomechanically stronger at time zero with:
  - More core sutures crossing repair site (*this is the most important factor*); minimum four-strand repairs are required for an early active motion rehabilitation protocol.
  - Larger core-suture diameter, ideally a 3–0 or 4–0 braided, nonabsorbable.
  - Increased distance from tendon end to transverse component of core suture.
    - 0.7 to 1.2 cm from the cut end of the tendon.
  - Locking stitch which is superior to a grasping stitch.
  - Dorsal placement of core suture which increases the strength of the repair.
  - Epitendinous suture which increases repair strength, decreases repair-site bulk, and decreases gap formation.
    - Epitendinous suture should be 2 mm deep and 2 mm from the cut end, circumferential.
    - If gap is >3 mm, the repair will *not* get stronger over time.

V. Surgical Technique

A. Basic Principles

- Repair within 7 to 10 day. If longer, the tendon retracts and can scar in, requiring a more extensive dissection and/or further trimming of cut ends.
- No-touch technique to minimize tendon adhesion formation (extrinsic healing). Use toothless forceps to hold tendon when passing sutures and minimize amount of tendon-grasping.

- Approach via a volar zig-zag (Bruner) or midaxial incision in digits. Identify neurovascular bundles and raise full-thickness flaps over tendon sheath.
- For access to cut tendon, elevate a window at the level of the cruciate pulleys (C1). If needed, can elevate C1, A3, and C2 as an entire window.
- If the tendon has retracted, use a pediatric feeding tube for retrieval, tying tendon to end with a grasping stitch for passage under A2. Once tendon stump is at level for repair, can stabilize stump with perpendicular 22-gauge needle.

B. Sutures

- Core
  - Four- to six-strand repair, need four-strand to start early active motion.
  - 3–0 or 4–0 suture (typically nonabsorbable, braided suture).
  - Ideal suture technique debatable (i.e., cruciate, modified Kessler, Winters-Gelberman, M-Tang, etc.).
- Epitendinous
  - 6–0 nonabsorbable monofilament suture, running (locking or nonlocking), circumferential.
  - Increases strength of repair by up to 300%.

C. Complications

- Reoperation rate = 6%.
- Rupture = 4%.
- Adhesions = 4%.

D. Recent Advances in Technique

- Wide-awake local anesthetic (WALANT) to test active strength, gapping, and gliding of tendon following repair (Lalonde, 2009):
  - Perform extension–flexion test to visualize tendon gliding beneath pulleys and determine if venting of pulleys is critical for gliding.
- Bulky repair site
  - Tension across the core suture is important for gap resistance (Wu and Tang, 2012). Allowing a certain degree of bulkiness at repair site (up to 120–130% of diameter of normal tendon) allows increased tension (Tang et al, 2017).
- Pulley release/venting
  - Venting of *part* of A2 or *all* of A4 may be key for tendon gliding.
  - Anatomic bowstringing is not equal to clinical functional loss flexion.

VI. Rehabilitation

- Transition over the past three decades from Kleinert or Duran passive protocols to controlled active motion (CAM) protocols.
- Basic principles
  - Information to include for therapist: Tendon repair quality, number of core suture strands (>4 strands across repair site needed to begin active motion protocol), epitendinous repair, and associated injuries (nerve, bone, and vascular).

- Early initiation of therapy, around day 5 (when gliding resistance is decreased), with slow and controlled motion even in the setting of edema (altering frequency, range of motion [ROM], and speed).
- Synergistic motion creates highest amount of flexor tendon gliding and differential excursion with low passive force.
- Active motion postoperative protocols
  - Early active motion
    - Dorsal block splint with wrist in extension, MCPs flexed.
    - Place-and-hold flexion, active extension within splint; tenodesis of wrist and digit out of splint for 4 weeks.
  - *Saint John Protocol* (Lalonde, 2016)
    - Immediate dorsal blocking splint with wrist in extension, MPs flexed.
    - Passive ROM warm-up, then active flexion to mid-range; "move it but you can't use it".
  - Nantong Protocol (Tang, 2007)
    - Wear dorsal blocking splint with flexion of wrist (20–30°) and MCPs (40–50°), IPs extended for 2.5 weeks, with active digital flexion through one-half to two-thirds motion.
    - At 2.5 weeks, transition new splint with wrist extension (30°), MCPs in flexion (40–50°), for 2.5 more weeks, with full passive flexion and still two-thirds of full motion.
  - Newer literature: Manchester short splint (Peck et al, 2014)
    - Postoperative splint that crosses wrist, allows 45 degrees extension and full wrist flexion.
    - Showed less flexion contracture at proximal interphalangeal (PIP) and greater flexion arc at distal interphalangeal (DIP) at 6 and 12 weeks (relative to forearm splint).
- Treatment progression
  - Depends on adhesion formation:
    - If limited, progress treatment.
    - If gliding is appropriate, protect.

VII. Reconstruction

A. Indications

- Failed zone II tendon repairs and chronic flexor tendon injuries.
- Options
  - Single-stage reconstruction with graft (use of palmaris, plantaris, or other FDS):
    - Pulley system must be intact.
    - Rarely indicated.
  - Two-stage approach
    - First stage: Silicone rod (typically 4 mm) placed; pulley reconstruction if necessary. Rod attached to distal stump of FDP or to distal phalanx over button.
    - If performing Paneva-Holevich, sew FDP to FDS just distal to lumbrical origin.
    - Second stage at 2 to 3 months: Palmaris, plantaris, or toe extensor. For the Paneva-Holevich, FDS is transected in Zone 5 and combine FDS/FDP graft is secured to distal phalanx.
- Outcomes are inferior to primary repair.

VIII. Summary

- Meticulous surgical approach, delicate tendon handling, multi-strand core repair with epitendinous suture, intraoperative mobilization with WALANT, and early CAM therapy protocols all contribute to obtaining the best outcome in flexor tendon. surgery.

Suggested Readings

Beredjiklian PK. Biologic aspects of flexor tendon laceration and repair. J Bone Joint Surg Am. 2003; 85(3):539–550

Doyle JR. Anatomy of the flexor tendon sheath and pulley system: a current review. J Hand Surg Am. 1989; 14(2 Pt 2):349–351

Dy CJ, Daluiski A, Do HT, Hernandez-Soria A, Marx R, Lyman S. The epidemiology of reoperation after flexor tendon repair. J Hand Surg Am. 2012; 37(5):919–924

Fufa DT, Osei DA, Calfee RP, Silva MJ, Thomopoulos S, Gelberman RH. The effect of core and epitendinous suture modifications on repair of intrasynovial flexor tendons in an in vivo canine model. J Hand Surg Am. 2012; 37 (12):2526–2531

Higgins A, Lalonde DH. Flexor tendon repair postoperative rehabilitation: the Saint John protocol. Plast Reconstr Surg Glob Open. 2016;4(11):e1134

Higgins A, Lalonde DH, Bell M, McKee D, Lalonde JF. Avoiding flexor tendon repair rupture with intraoperative total active movement examination. Plast Reconstr Surg. 2010; 126(3):941–945

Lalonde DH. Wide-awake flexor tendon repair. Plast Reconstr Surg. 2009; 123(2):623–625

Lalonde DH, Martin AL. Wide-awake flexor tendon repair and early tendon mobilization in zones 1 and 2. Hand Clin. 2013; 29(2):207–213

Lundborg G. Experimental flexor tendon healing without adhesion formation—a new concept of tendon nutrition and intrinsic healing mechanisms. A preliminary report. Hand. 1976; 8(3):235–238

Matarrese MR, Hammert WC. Flexor tendon rehabilitation. J Hand Surg Am. 2012; 37(11):2386–2388

Moore T, Anderson B, Seiler JG, III. Flexor tendon reconstruction. J Hand Surg Am. 2010; 35(6):1025–1030

Peck FH, Roe AE, Ng CY, Duff C, McGrouther DA, Lees VC. The Manchester short splint: a change to splinting practice in the rehabilitation of zone II flexor tendon repairs. Hand Ther. 2014; 19(2):47–53

Sourmelis SG, McGrouther DA. Retrieval of the retracted flexor tendon. J Hand Surg [Br]. 1987; 12(1):109–111

Strickland JW. Development of flexor tendon surgery: twenty-five years of progress. J Hand Surg Am. 2000; 25 (2):214–235

Tang JB. Indications, methods, postoperative motion and outcome evaluation of primary flexor tendon repairs in Zone 2. J Hand Surg Eur Vol. 2007; 32(2):118–129

Tang JB. Release of the A4 pulley to facilitate zone II flexor tendon repair. J Hand Surg Am. 2014; 39(11):2300–2307

Tang JB, Zhang Y, Cao Y, Xie RG. Core suture purchase affects strength of tendon repairs. J Hand Surg Am. 2005; 30 (6):1262–1266

Tang JB, Zhou X, Pan ZJ, Qing J, Gong KT, Chen J. Strong digital flexor tendon repair, extension-flexion test, and early active flexion: experience in 300 tendons. Hand Clin. 2017; 33(3):455–463

Trumble TE, Vedder NB, Seiler JG, III, Hanel DP, Diao E, Pettrone S. Zone-II flexor tendon repair: a randomized prospective trial of active place-and-hold therapy compared with passive motion therapy. J Bone Joint Surg Am. 2010; 92(6):1381–1389

Winters SC, Gelberman RH, Woo SL, Chan SS, Grewal R, Seiler JG, III. The effects of multiple-strand suture methods on the strength and excursion of repaired intrasynovial flexor tendons: a biomechanical study in dogs. J Hand Surg Am. 1998; 23(1):97–104

Wu YF, Tang JB. Effects of tension across the tendon repair site on tendon gap and ultimate strength. J Hand Surg Am. 2012; 37(5):906–912

Wu YF, Tang JB. Recent developments in flexor tendon repair techniques and factors influencing strength of the tendon repair. J Hand Surg Eur Vol. 2014; 39(1):6–19

15 Extensor Tendon Injury, Repair, and Reconstruction

Viviana Serra López, Adnan N. Cheema, and David J. Bozentka

Abstract

Extensor tendons are susceptible to injury because of their superficial location. Along with ligamentous structures and intrinsic musculature, they provide stability to the different articulations of the hand and allow for range of motion. Extensor tendon injuries are classified based their location (Zones I–VIII), with each zone having its own characteristic presentations and management. Diagnosis is usually clinical, with various imaging modalities available as adjuncts. Treatment may be nonoperative or surgical, depending on injury zone and chronicity. Primary repair is performed when the gap needed to bridge is small. Certain suture techniques have been shown to be superior in each injury zone, taking into consideration the increasing thickness of the extensor tendons as the injury becomes more proximal. Reconstruction techniques are varied, depending on injury zone and surgeon's preference and can be used in cases where primary repair is not feasible. Postinjury rehabilitation options include early active mobilization and dynamic splinting regimens, which are important to avoid complications such as adhesions, loss of range of motion, and tendon shortening.

Keywords: Extensor tendon injury, central slip, boutonniere deformity, tendon reconstruction

I. Introduction

- Traumatic tendon injuries to the hand can have an incidence of 33 injuries per 100,000 person-years, with up to 85% involving an extensor tendon.[1]
- Studies suggest that when a laceration is encountered in the dorsum of hand, there is a 50% chance of finding a concomitant tendon injury.[2]

II. Anatomy

A. Extrinsic Extensor Muscles

- Originate in the elbow and forearm.
- Superficial group: Extensor carpi radialis longus (ECRL), extensor carpi radialis brevis (ECRB), extensor digitorum communis (EDC), extensor digiti minimi (EDM), and extensor carpi ulnaris (ECU).
- Deep group: Abductor pollicis longus (APL), extensor pollicis brevis (EPB), extensor pollicis longus (EPL), and extensor indicis proprius (EIP).
- ECRL is innervated by the radial nerve, ECRB innervated by the posterior interosseous nerve (PIN) or superficial radial sensory nerve,[3,4] and the remaining muscles by the PIN.
- Extrinsic extensor muscle tendons travel through six compartments in the dorsal aspect of the wrist, covered by the extensor retinaculum (▶ Fig. 15.1).
  - First compartment: APL and EPB tendons.

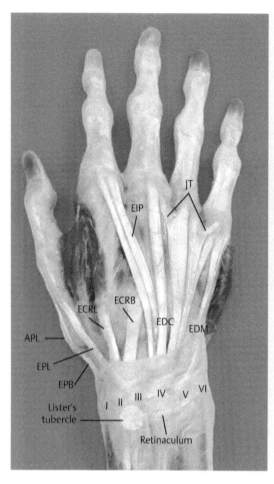

Fig. 15.1 Extensor tendon compartments at the level of the wrist, covered by the extensor retinaculum. Compartments are numbered I to VI from radial to ulnar. Lister's tubercle separates compartments II and III. APL, abductor pollicis longus; ECRB, extensor carpi radialis brevis; EDC, extensor digitorum communis; EDM, extensor digiti minimi; ECRL, Extensor carpi radialis longus; EIP, extensor indicis proprius; EPB, extensor pollicis brevis; EPL, extensor pollicis longus; and JT, juncturae tendinum. Used with permission from Bo Tang J, Amadio PC, Guimberteau JC, Chang J, eds. Tendon Surgery of the Hand. 1st ed. Philadelphia, PA: Elsevier; 2012:10.

- Second compartment: ECRL and ECRB tendons, with ECRB located ulnar to ECRL.
- Third compartment: EPL.
- Fourth compartment: Four tendons of EDC and EIP tendon.
  - EIP is commonly located ulnar to the index finger EDC.
  - Contains terminal branch of PIN, which provides sensory and proprioceptive fibers to dorsal wrist capsule.
- Fifth compartment: EDM.
- Sixth compartment: ECU.

B. Intrinsic Muscles

- Originate and insert within the hand.
  - Four lumbrical muscles, numbered sequentially from radial to ulnar:
    - Originate from flexor digitorum profundus tendons.
    - Insert onto the lateral band on the radial side of each proximal phalanx.

- First and second lumbricals are innervated by the median nerve, third and fourth lumbricals are innervated by the ulnar nerve.
- Function is to flex metacarpophalangeal (MCP) joints and extend interphalangeal (IP) joints.
  ○ Seven interossei muscles: Three palmar interossei and four dorsal interossei:
    - Originate from the metacarpals.
    - Insert onto the proximal phalanges and extensor expansions.
    - Innervated by the ulnar nerve.
    - Function is to abduct and adduct the fingers.

C. Tendons

- Extrinsic tendons run over MCP joints, then trifurcate into a central slip and two lateral slips:
  ○ The central slip inserts at the base of the middle phalanx.
  ○ The lateral slips insert at the base of the distal phalanx as a single terminal extensor tendon.
- Intrinsic tendons form lateral bands on each side of the digits, which join the extensor mechanism just proximal to the proximal interphalangeal (PIP) joints (▶ Fig. 15.2).

D. Additional Stabilizers

- Juncturae tendinum: Interconnect EDC tendons proximal to the MCP joints.
- Sagittal bands: Form a sling around the extensor tendons to maintain their central position, attaching them to the volar plate at the level of the MCP joints.
- Transverse retinacular ligaments: Prevent dorsal subluxation of the conjoined lateral bands at the level of the PIP joint.
  ○ Disruption results in swan neck deformity: PIP hyperextension with distal interphalangeal (DIP) flexion.

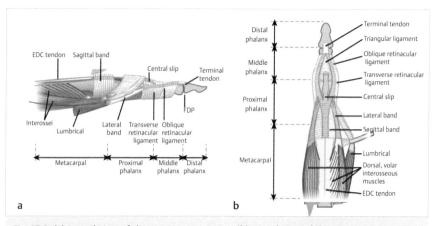

Fig. 15.2 (a) Lateral view of the extensor apparatus. **(b)** Dorsal view of the extensor apparatus. Used with permission from Wolfe S, Hotchkiss R, eds. Green's Operative Hand Surgery, 2-Volume Set. 7th ed. Philadelphia, PA: Elsevier; 2016:155.

- Triangular ligament: Prevents volar subluxation of the conjoined lateral bands by connecting them at the level of the middle phalanx.
  - Disruption results in boutonniere deformity: PIP flexion and hyperextension of the DIP.
- Oblique retinacular ligaments: Coordinate PIP and DIP joint movements.[5]

III. Injury Zones

A. Location

- Injury zones are based on location, as described by Kleinert and Verdan (▶ Fig. 15.3).[6]
- Zone I: DIP joint. Injuries are further categorized based on Doyle's classification[7]:
  - Type 1: Closed, with or without avulsion fracture (most common pattern).
  - Type 2: Open injury.
  - Type 3: Open injury with loss of soft tissue coverage and tendon substance.
  - Type 4:
    - Type 4a: Transepiphyseal fracture in children.
    - Type 4b: Phalanx base fracture involving 20 to 50% of articular surface.
    - Type 4c: Phalanx base fracture involving 50% or more of articular surface.
- Zone II: Middle phalanx.
- Zone III: PIP joint.
- Zone IV: Proximal phalanx.

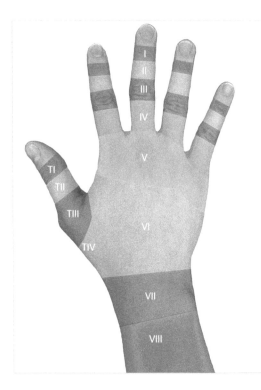

Fig. 15.3 Extensor tendon injury zones as described by Kleinert and Verdan.

- Zone V: MCP joint.
  - Sagittal band injuries occur at this level and can be classified into three types[8]:
    - Type 1: Contusion with no tendon tear.
    - Type 2: Tendon subluxation.
    - Type 3: Dislocation of tendon between metacarpal heads.
- Zone VI: Dorsal hand.
- Zone VII: Dorsal retinaculum.
  - Tendon ruptures may also present in association with rheumatoid arthritis:
    - Vaughan-Jackson syndrome: Rupture of extensor tendons resulting from dorsal ulnar head prominence, affecting EDM tendon first and proceeding radially.
    - Caput ulna syndrome: Synovitis in distal radioulnar joint leads to capsular and ECU sheath stretching with ECU volar subluxation, eventually leading to a prominent ulna causing additional stress over the already weakened tendons.
- Zone VIII: Distal third of the forearm.

B. Thumb

- Zones are similarly defined:
  - Zone TI: IP joint.
  - Zone TII: Proximal phalanx.
  - Zone TIII: MP joint.
  - Zone TIV: First metacarpal.

IV. Presentation and Physical Examination

- Obtain detailed history including injury mechanism and position of digit during injury.
- Open injuries warrant complete neurovascular examination.
- Completely severed extensor tendons may present with finger in flexion.
- Digits should be examined individually to eliminate any contributions from other tendons, with passive range of motion and active range of motion against resistance in order to identify partial lacerations and any extensor lag.
- Tenodesis examination can be performed: Normally, passive wrist extension results in the digits held in flexion and passive wrist flexion results in the digits held in extension.
  - Extensor tendon injury may result in decreased passive finger extension when ranging from wrist extension to wrist flexion.
- Two-point discrimination can be used to assess for sensory deficits, which is normal if less than 5 mm in the volar aspect of the digits.

A. Zone-Specific Presentations

- Zone I: Mallet finger deformity (flexion of DIP joint), with an injury mechanism of forced flexion during active extension.
- Zones II and IV: Usually arise secondary to a laceration.
- Zone III: Central slip disruption results in PIP extension weakness and eventual boutonniere deformity with volar migration of lateral bands (▶ Fig. 15.4).
  - Elson's test can be performed to evaluate the integrity of the central slip:
    - Position the patient's PIP in 90 degrees of flexion with the purpose of keeping the central slip taut. The patient is asked to extend DIP while the provider applies

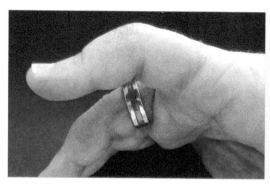

Fig. 15.4 Classic physical examination finding in boutonniere deformity. The proximal interphalangeal (PIP) joint is flexed, and the distal interphalangeal (DIP) is hyperextended. Used with permission from Boyer MI, Chang J, eds. 100 Hand Cases. New York, NY: Thieme, 2016:217.

force to the middle phalanx. Test is abnormal if DIP extends via the action of the lateral bands.

- Zone V: Open tendon injuries often result from striking someone in the mouth with a clenched fist, whereas sagittal band ruptures are associated with resisted extension of the finger (flicking motion).
  - Sagittal band injury: Patient cannot actively extend the MCP joint from a fully flexed position, but can hold in the MCP joint in extension once finger is passively extended.
  - Type 2 sagittal band injuries may present with snapping at the MCP joint with flexion and extension due to tendon subluxation.
  - Type 3 injuries may result in ulnar deviation if radial sagittal bands are involved.
- Zone VI: Challenging to determine deficits via physical examination if juncta tendinae is intact.
- Zone VII: Patient may present with an extensor tendon rupture following a history of distal radius fracture treated with a volar plate with prominent dorsal screws, or a minimally displaced distal radius fracture leading to EPL rupture.
- Zone VIII: Usually patient has a history of open trauma or hardware complications, with closed injuries being rare.

V. Imaging Modalities

- Diagnosis is most often made by clinical examination alone. When necessary, diagnostic imaging is based mostly on MRI or ultrasound.
- MRI
  - Hyperintense signal at site of tear or surrounding tissue on T2-weighted imaging is usually first sign of abnormality.[9]
  - Signal may be intermediate if scarring is present, as in chronic injuries.
- Ultrasound
  - Partial ruptures characterized by hypoechoic sections of tendon or by swelling and effusion.
  - Complete ruptures characterized by absence of the tendon in its anatomical location or by visualizing a gap.
  - Dynamic ultrasound has a role in sagittal band injuries (Zone V), where extensor tendon subluxation or dislocation can be visualized while the patient performs flexion and extension of the involved finger.[10]

A. Other Imaging Modalities

- Radiographs
  - X-rays should be performed to evaluate for associated bony injuries or retained foreign bodies.
  - May reveal pathologic conditions associated with chronic injuries.
    - Rheumatoid arthritis commonly presents with ulnar deviation of MCP joints.
- Role of CT is limited in tendon injuries.

VI. Treatment

A. Nonoperative Treatment

- Zone I: Most common indication for nonoperative treatment is closed injury, and fracture fragment involving less than one-third of the joint surface area.[11]
  - DIP joint is immobilized in an extension splint.
  - Most studies have found no differences in DIP joint extension deficits when comparing different types of splints.[11]
- Zone II: Partial injuries that involve 50% or less of the tendon and show no extensor lag or weakness may undergo splinting for 1 to 2 weeks.
- Zone III: Acute central slip injuries may undergo extension splinting of the PIP joint for 6 weeks, with DIP joint flexion exercises performed concurrently, followed by 4 to 6 weeks of night splinting.
- Zone IV: If there is no loss of PIP joint extension, the injury can be treated with splinting and early motion.
- Zone V: Splinting has been successful in both traumatic and atraumatic sagittal band incompetence using a sagittal band bridge or yoke splint.[12]

B. Operative Treatment via Primary Repair

- Repair should generally be performed within 1 to 2 weeks from injury.
- Zone I: Most common surgical indications are involvement of more than one-third of the articular surface, subluxation of distal phalanx, and failure of nonoperative treatment.[11]
  - Most surgical techniques involve use of K-wire fixation across the DIP joint.
- Zone II: Complete tendon injuries should be repaired primarily and supplemented with K-wire fixation if needed.
- Zone III: Primary repair is indicated in open injuries, displaced avulsion fractures, and with PIP instability.
  - Open lacerations often require primary repair.
  - Avulsions and distal central slip injuries may be treated with suture anchors.[13]
- Zone IV: A loss of active extension warrants surgical exploration.
  - Cadaveric study comparing different suture techniques found that the Modified Becker was the strongest in this zone (▶ Fig. 15.5).[14]
- Zone VI: Cadaveric study comparing three repairs found that a running-interlocking horizontal mattress repair resulted in more stiffness of the construct and less tendon shortening (▶ Fig. 15.6).[15]
- Zone VII: Typically involve damage to extensor retinaculum, which is released to improve visualization.
  - Repair of tendons at this level should be performed with core suture.[13]

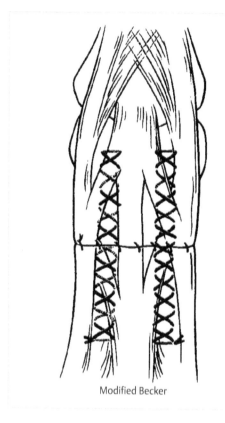

Modified Becker

Fig. 15.5 Schematic diagram of a Modified Becker suture for Zone IV tendon repairs. Criss-cross suture is placed on each side of the injured tendon with a running epitenon suture. Used with permission from Woo SH, Tsai TM, Kleinert HE, Chew WYC, Voor MJ. A biomechanical comparison of four extensor tendon repair techniques in zone IV. Plast Reconstr Surg 2005:1676.

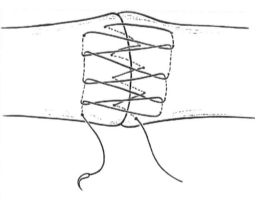

Fig. 15.6 Running-interlocking horizontal mattress repair technique: simple running suture begins at the near end, followed by an interlocking horizontal mattress suture which starts at the far end. Used with permission from Lee SK, Dubey A, Kim BH, Zingman A, Landa J, Paksima N. A biomechanical study of extensor tendon repair methods: introduction to the running-interlocking horizontal mattress extensor tendon repair technique. J Hand Surg 2010:21.

C. Operative Treatment via Reconstruction

- Tendon lengthening may be performed to bridge small gaps, especially in proximal lesions.
  - Techniques include Z-plasties and V-Y plasties proximal to the zone of trauma.[16]

- Primary repair in Zones II and IV is limited because the gaps cannot be easily bridged.
  - Local tendon flaps have been successful for repairs in Zones II and IV when the remaining tendon proximal to the defect is at least the length of the defect plus an additional 0.5 cm.[17]
- Zone III: Central slip reconstruction can be performed in chronic deformities, with a variety of available techniques:
  - Terminal tenotomy to improve DIP flexion.
  - Central slip advancement.
  - Autograft for central slip deficiency or flexor digitorum superficialis slip via bone tunnel.[18]
  - Central slip turndown.[19]
  - Lateral band mobilization.[20]
- Zone V: If a patient cannot undergo primary repair after failing nonoperative treatment, reconstruction of the sagittal band can be performed using a distally based slip of EDC around the collateral ligament or dynamic transfer of lumbrical muscles.[21]
- Zone VI: EIP tendon transfer commonly performed for EPL ruptures.[22]
  - Chronic injuries may require side-to-side tendon transfers or tendon grafts.
- Zone VII: Chronic tears require tendon transfer or grafting.[13]

VII. Postoperative Rehabilitation Protocols

- Early motion is encouraged to limit adhesion formation and is considered if repair has adequate strength, highlighting the importance of using mechanically robust constructs.
- Static splinting has been associated with worse functional outcomes.[23]
- Early range of motion regimens developed to improve outcomes:
  - For patients who underwent repairs in Zones V to VII, no differences were found at long-term follow-up in range of motion when comparing static versus dynamic splinting while undergoing rehabilitation exercise programs.[24]
- For Zones I and II, encourage PIP and MCP motion while keeping DIP splinted in extension for at least 6 weeks following primary repair.

VIII. Complications

- Range of motion limitations: Can result from tendon shortening or adhesions.
  - A study following long-term results of repaired extensor tendon injuries noted that there was in fact greater loss of finger flexion than loss of extension.[23]
  - In distal injuries, tendon length is very sensitive to length changes, with 1 mm shortening in the terminal tendon leading to severe loss of DIP joint flexion.[25]
  - Tenodesis restraint can result from tendon shortening or scarring, further limiting the ability to regain range of motion.
  - Tenolysis may be performed if nonoperative management fails and there is no loss of tendon length.
  - Tendon release can be performed if there is loss of tendon length.
- Deformities can result from untreated injuries:
  - Mallet finger, swan neck deformity, and boutonniere deformity.

References

[1] de Jong JP, Nguyen JT, Sonnema AJM, Nguyen EC, Amadio PC, Moran SL. The incidence of acute traumatic tendon injuries in the hand and wrist: a 10-year population-based study. Clin Orthop Surg. 2014; 6(2):196–202

[2] Tuncali D, Yavuz N, Terzioglu A, Aslan G. The rate of upper-extremity deep-structure injuries through small penetrating lacerations. Ann Plast Surg. 2005; 55(2):146–148

[3] Dhall U, Kanta S. Variations in the nerve supply to extensor carpi radialis brevis. J Anat Soc India. 2001; 50 (2):134–136

[4] Cricenti SV, Deangelis MA, Didio LJA, Ebraheim NA, Rupp RE, Didio AS. Innervation of the extensor carpi radialis brevis and supinator muscles: levels of origin and penetration of these muscular branches from the posterior interosseous nerve. J Shoulder Elbow Surg. 1994; 3(6):390–394

[5] Adkinson JM, Johnson SP, Chung KC. The clinical implications of the oblique retinacular ligament. J Hand Surg Am. 2014; 39(3):535–541

[6] Kleinert HE, Verdan C. Report of the Committee on Tendon Injuries (International Federation of Societies for Surgery of the Hand). J Hand Surg Am. 1983; 8(5 Pt 2):794–798

[7] Strauch RJ. Extensor tendon injury. In: Wolfe SW, Hotchkiss RN, Pederson WC, Kozin SH, Choen MS, eds. Green's Operative Hand Surgery, 2-Volume Set. 7th ed. Philadelphia: Elsevier; 2016:152–182

[8] Rayan GM, Murray D. Classification and treatment of closed sagittal band injuries. J Hand Surg Am. 1994; 19 (4):590–594

[9] Weinreb JH, Sheth C, Apostolakos J, et al. Tendon structure, disease, and imaging. Muscles Ligaments Tendons J. 2014; 4(1):66–73

[10] Lee SA, Kim BH, Kim S-J, Kim JN, Park S-Y, Choi K. Current status of ultrasonography of the finger. Ultrasonography. 2016; 35(2):110–123

[11] Lin JS, Samora JB. Surgical and nonsurgical management of mallet finger: a systematic review. J Hand Surg Am. 2018; 43(2):146–163.e2

[12] Peelman J, Markiewitz A, Kiefhaber T, Stern P. Splintage in the treatment of sagittal band incompetence and extensor tendon subluxation. J Hand Surg Eur Vol. 2015; 40(3):287–290

[13] Matzon JL, Bozentka DJ. Extensor tendon injuries. J Hand Surg Am. 2010; 35(5):854–861

[14] Woo S-H, Tsai T-M, Kleinert HE, Chew WYC, Voor MJ. A biomechanical comparison of four extensor tendon repair techniques in zone IV. Plast Reconstr Surg. 2005; 115(6):1674–1681, discussion 1682–1683

[15] Lee SK, Dubey A, Kim BH, Zingman A, Landa J, Paksima N. A biomechanical study of extensor tendon repair methods: introduction to the running-interlocking horizontal mattress extensor tendon repair technique. J Hand Surg Am. 2010; 35(1):19–23

[16] Schubert CD, Giunta RE. Extensor tendon repair and reconstruction. Clin Plast Surg. 2014; 41(3):525–531

[17] Kochevar A, Rayan G, Angel M. Extensor tendon reconstruction for zones II and IV using local tendon flap: a cadaver study. J Hand Surg Am. 2009; 34(7):1269–1275

[18] Patel SS, Singh N, Clark C, Stone J, Nydick J. Reconstruction of traumatic central slip injuries: technique using a slip of flexor digitorum superficialis. Tech Hand Up Extrem Surg. 2018; 22(4):150–155

[19] Snow JW. A method for reconstruction of the central slip of the extensor tendon of a finger. Plast Reconstr Surg. 1976; 57(4):455–459

[20] Aiache A, Barsky AJ, Weiner DL. Prevention of the boutonniere deformity. Plast Reconstr Surg. 1970; 46 (2):164–167

[21] Segalman KA. Dynamic lumbrical muscle transfer for correction of posttraumatic extensor tendon subluxation. Tech Hand Up Extrem Surg. 2006; 10(2):107–113

[22] Magnussen PA, Harvey FJ, Tonkin MA. Extensor indicis proprius transfer for rupture of the extensor pollicis longus tendon. J Bone Joint Surg Br. 1990; 72(5):881–883

[23] Newport ML, Blair WF, Steyers CM, Jr. Long-term results of extensor tendon repair. J Hand Surg Am. 1990; 15 (6):961–966

[24] Chester DL, Beale S, Beveridge L, Nancarrow JD, Titley OG. A prospective, controlled, randomized trial comparing early active extension with passive extension using a dynamic splint in the rehabilitation of repaired extensor tendons. J Hand Surg [Br]. 2002; 27(3):283–288

[25] Schweitzer TP, Rayan GM. The terminal tendon of the digital extensor mechanism: Part II, kinematic study. J Hand Surg Am. 2004; 29(5):903–908

16 Peripheral Nerve Injuries and Repair and Reconstruction

Suresh K. Nayar and John Ingari

Abstract

In this segment, we focus on peripheral nerve injury and repair/reconstruction. Nerves are encased in epineurium which contains fascicles sheathed in perineurium. Fascicles contain individual nerve fibers. Nerves can be injured from stretching, compression, or laceration. Nerve regeneration is slow and is affected by patient age, level of injury, injury pattern, and timing of repair. An electromyogram is the first primary test to assess nerve function and other imaging modalities, such as MR neurography, can better characterize injury patterns. Nonoperative treatment is indicated for neuropraxia and axonotmesis while neurorrhaphy, nerve grafting, conduits, and transfers can be considered for more severe injury.

Keywords: Peripheral nerve injury, peripheral nerve reconstruction, peripheral nerve repair, peripheral nerve grafting, peripheral nerve transfers

I. Anatomy

- Peripheral nerves originate from brachial plexus with separate sensory (▸ Fig. 16.1) and muscle innervation (▸ Fig. 16.2).
- Characteristic nerve course throughout upper extremity (▸ Fig. 16.3).
- Structure (▸ Fig. 16.4).
  - Epineurium—dense external sheath of connective tissue which contains fascicles.
  - Fascicles are surrounded by perineurium which encompasses nerve fibers which are each individually encased in endoneurium.

II. Mechanism of Injury

A. Stretching

- Stretching by > 8% can diminish a nerve's blood supply.
- Stretching by >15% can disrupt axons.
- Axonal transport stops after 15 minutes of ischemia, recovers if restored within 12 to 24 hours.
- Common injury patterns
  - Brachial plexus
    - "Stingers," brachial plexus stretch with violent contralateral neck flexion.
  - Axillary
    - Humeral head compression during extreme abduction.
    - Humeral surgical neck fracture.
    - Direct compression through axilla.
    - Shoulder dislocation.
    - Compression in quadrilateral space.
    - Prolonged use of crutches.

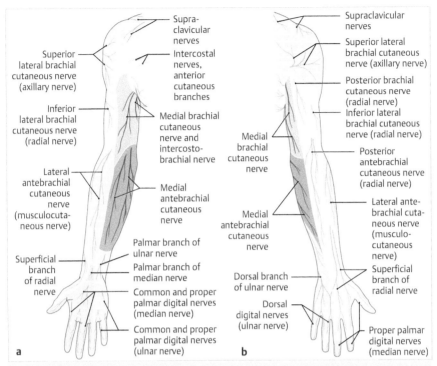

Fig. 16.1 Sensory distribution of upper extremity peripheral nerves. **(a)** Anterior view, **(b)** posterior view. Source: THIEME Atlas of Anatomy, Volume 1: General Anatomy and Musculoskeletal System. 3rd ed. Thieme; 2020. Illustration by Karl Wesker/Markus Voll.

- Long thoracic
  - Violent traction.
  - Shoulder depression with contralateral neck flexion.
  - Prolonged compression (backpacker's palsy).
- Suprascapular
  - Entrapment under transverse scapular splinoglenoid ligaments.
  - Trauma to scapular spine.
- Median
  - Trauma within pronator teres, under flexor digitorum superficialis, or to carpal tunnel.
  - Elbow dislocation (▶ Fig. 16.5).
- Musculocutaneous
  - Shoulder dislocation.
  - Coracobrachialis hypertrophy.
- Radial
  - Proximal or midshaft humerus fracture.
  - Proximal radius fracture.
  - Trauma to supinator, affecting posterior interosseous nerve (PIN).
- Ulnar
  - Injury to cubital tunnel or Guyon's canal.

Cervical nerve root:	C5	C6	C7	C8	T1
Musculocutaneous	Biceps				
	Brachialis				
	Coracobrachialis				
Axillary	Deltoid				
	Teres minor				
Radial		Triceps			
		Brachioradialis			
		Anconeus			
		Extensor carpi radialis longus			
Deep branch		Supinator			
		Extensor carpi radialis brevis			
PIN			Extensor carpi ulnaris		
			Extensor digitorum		
			Extensor pollicis longus and brevis		
			Extensor indicis		
			Extensor digiti minimi		
			Abductor pollicus longus		
Median			Pronator teres		
			Flexor carpi radialis		
			Palmaris longus		
			Flexor digitorum superficialis		
			Lumbricals (middle and index)		
			Opponens pollicis		
			Abductor pollicis brevis		
			Flexor pollicis brevis		
AIN			Flexor pollicus longus		
			Pronator quadratus		
			Flexor digitorum profundus (middle and index)		
Ulnar				Flexor carpi ulnaris	
				Flexor digitorum profundus (ring and little)	
				Opponens digiti minimi	
				Flexor digiti minimi brevis	
				Abductor digiti minimi	
				Interossei	
				Lumbricals (ring and little)	
				Adductor pollicis	

Fig. 16.2 Muscle innervation of upper extremity peripheral nerves. Colored muscle groups correspond to primary cervical nerve root.

B. Compression or Crush-Induced Ischemia

- Local deformation causes fiber ischemia and increased vascular permeability.
- Increased edema interferes with axon transport and nerve function.
- Persistent injury can lead to fibrosis.
- Tissue pressures:
  - ≤ 30 mm Hg = paresthesia and increased nerve latency.
  - ≥ 30 mm Hg = nerve conduction blocked.

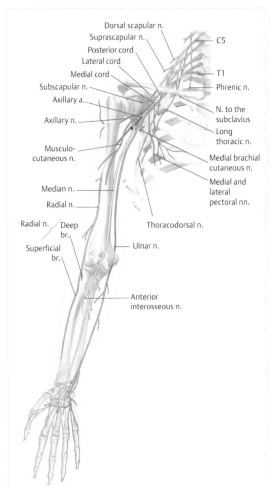

Dorsal scapular n.
Suprascapular n.
Posterior cord
Lateral cord
Medial cord
Subscapular n.
Axillary a.
Axillary n.
Musculo-
cutaneous n.
Median n.
Radial n.
Radial n. Deep br.
Superficial br.
C5
T1
Phrenic n.
N. to the subclavius
Long thoracic n.
Medial brachial cutaneous n.
Medial and lateral pectoral nn.
Thoracodorsal n.
Ulnar n.
Anterior interosseous n.

Fig. 16.3 Course of peripheral nerves. Source: Schünke M, Schulte E, Schumacher U et al, eds. THIEME Atlas of Anatomy, Volume 3: Head, Neck, and Neuroanatomy. 3rd ed. Thieme; 2020. Illustration by Karl Wesker/Markus Voll.

C. Laceration

• Sharp injury can lead to nerve end retraction and axonal degeneration.

III. Pathophysiology

A. Regeneration after Transection

• Distal nerve section degrades through Wallerian degeneration.
• At 1 month, proximal end begins to migrate toward distal segment at 1 mm/day.
• Local neurotrophic factors may aid in regrowth.
• After 12 months of denervation, a muscle is no longer receptive to reinnervation.

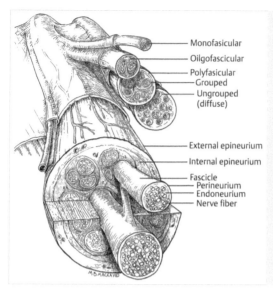

Fig. 16.4 Peripheral nerve illustration. Source: Wolfla C, Resnick D, eds. Neurosurgical Operative Atlas: Spine and Peripheral Nerves. 2nd ed. Thieme; 2007.

Monofasicular
Oilgofascicular
Polyfasicular
—Grouped
Ungrouped (diffuse)

External epineurium
Internal epineurium
Fascicle
Perineurium
Endoneurium
Nerve fiber

IV. Prognosis

- Successful recovery affected by:
  - Age (favorable in younger patients).
  - Level of injury (proximal injuries have worse prognosis).
  - Injury pattern (sharp transections recover better than crush or avulsion injuries).
  - Timing of repair (window of repair <12–18 months).
- Return of pain is first sign of recovery.
- Radial and musculocutaneous nerves have better recovery potential compared to median and ulnar.

V. Classification Systems

A. Seddon Classification

- Neuropraxia
  - Focal damage to myelin fibers around axons.
  - Typically reversible, improvement seen within days to weeks with near-complete resolution.
- Axonotmesis
  - Direct injury to axons with intact neural connective tissue.
  - No destruction of Schwann cells, perineurium, or epineurium.
  - Nerve regeneration possible but prolonged over several months often with incomplete recovery.
- Neurotmesis
  - Complete disruption of axon.
  - Low likelihood of clinical recovery.

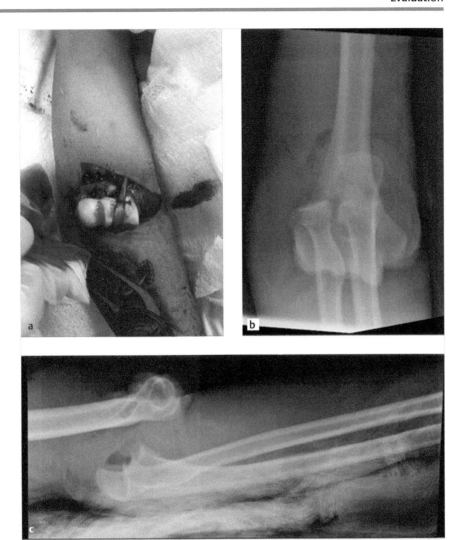

Fig. 16.5 Open anterior elbow dislocation with median nerve on stretch. (a) Opening of antecubital fossa with median nerve lying anterior over trochlea. (b) Anteroposterior (AP) and (c) lateral radiographs showing dislocation without fracture.

VI. Evaluation

- Electromyogram (EMG) and nerve conduction testing:
  - Primary test for peripheral nerve injury.
  - Assesses sensory and motor function and can detect level and severity of injury based on signal latency.
- Imaging
  - Magnetic resonance imaging (MRI):
    - Adjunct to EMG to assess for structural defect.
    - Can show chronic changes from muscle denervation (e.g., fatty atrophy).

VII. Treatment

A. Nonoperative

- Observe with sequential EMG.
- Indicated for neuropraxia or axonotmesis.

B. Surgical Repair (Neurorrhaphy)

- Need well-vascularized repair bed with viable soft tissue coverage and skeletal stability.
- Nerve ends are sharply debrided of devitalized or scar tissue; fascicles matched as accurately as possible to avoid scar deposition.
- Need postoperative immobilization for ≥2 weeks.

C. Epineurial Repair

- Typically the most effective primary repair.
- Involves microsurgery instrumentation and technique.
- Use a fine monofilament suture (e.g., 9–0 nylon) and/or fibrin glue (▶ Fig. 16.6).

D. Fascicular Repair

- Fascicular approximation by perineurial repair (▶ Fig. 16.7 and ▶ Fig. 16.8).
- Used for median and ulnar nerve injuries in the distal third of forearm.
- More precise than epineurial repair but requires intraneural dissection which can cause increased scar formation.
- Outcomes similar to epineurial repair.

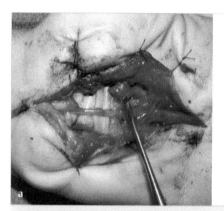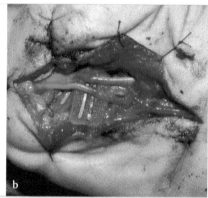

Fig. 16.6 Epineurial repair of median nerve in distal third of forearm using 9–0 nylon. **(a)** Freer elevator showing distal segment of transected nerve. **(b)** Repaired nerve, suture thickness only appreciated with microscopy. Courtesy of Dr. Ryan Katz (Curtis Hand Center, Union Memorial Hospital, Baltimore, MD).

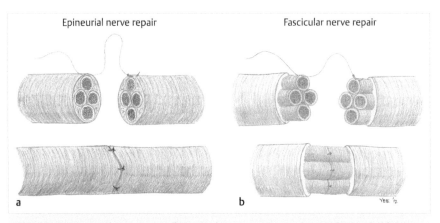

Fig. 16.7 (a) Epineurial nerve repair. (b) Fascicular nerve repair. Source: Mackinnon S, ed. Nerve Surgery. 1st ed. Thieme; 2015.

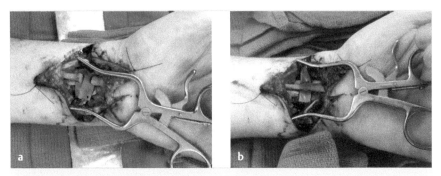

Fig. 16.8 (a, b) Fascicular repair of median nerve followed by epineurial repair. Courtesy of Dr. Laura Lewallen (Johns Hopkins Hospital, Baltimore, MD).

E. Nerve grafting

- Used when defect ≥2.5 cm (▶ Fig. 16.9), gold standard for injuries ≥5.0 cm.
- Type of autograft has no effect on recovery or function.
- Digital nerve defects:
  ○ Sural nerve for wrist defect, proximal to digital nerve bifurcation.
  ○ Lateral antebrachial cutaneous nerve for metacarpophalangeal (MCP) to distal interphalangeal (DIP) level.
  ○ Anterior interosseous nerve (AIN), PIN, or medial antebrachial cutaneous nerve at the level of DIP.

F. Conduits

- Collagen constructs supporting nutrient and neurotrophic factor transport.
- Used when defect is <2.0 cm.
- Similar results to autologous grafting when the gap is ≤5 mm.

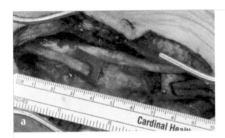
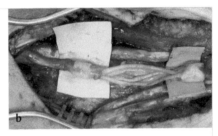
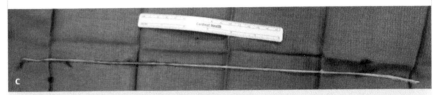

Fig. 16.9 (a–c) Median nerve repair with sural nerve autograft. Hanno-Millesi cable grafting technique. Courtesy of Dr. Ryan Katz (Curtis Hand Center, Union Memorial Hospital, Baltimore, MD).

G. Nerve Transfers

- Effective for injuries where grafting cannot be used (e.g., cervical nerve-root avulsion or large segmental nerve injuries).

Suggested Readings

Griffin JW, Hogan MV, Chhabra AB, Deal DN. Peripheral nerve repair and reconstruction. J Bone Joint Surg Am. 2013; 95(23):2144–2151

Grinsell D, Keating CP. Peripheral nerve reconstruction after injury: a review of clinical and experimental therapies. BioMed Res Int. 2014; 2014:698256

Lin MY, Manzano G, Gupta R. Nerve allografts and conduits in peripheral nerve repair. Hand Clin. 2013; 29(3):331–348

17 Nerve Palsies and Tendon/Nerve Transfers for Injuries at or Distal to the Elbow

Roshan T. Melvani and Aviram M. Giladi

Abstract
Tendon transfers are utilized to reestablish balance to a disabled, damaged, or devoid neuromuscular-motor unit. They are indicated for rejuvenation of muscular function after peripheral nerve damage, trauma to the brachial plexus or spinal cord, or irrecoverable injury to tendons/muscles. The goal is to equalize the surrounding musculotendinous forces and restore functional activity. Tendon transfers are most commonly used in the hand and forearm to address radial, median, or ulnar nerve dysfunction. Understanding the principles for transfer can ensure maximal benefit and optimize postoperative results. Nerve transfers may be an alternative option depending on the nature and chronicity of the injury.

Keywords: Tendon, transfer, brachial plexus, neuropathy, median nerve palsy, radial nerve palsy, ulnar nerve palsy, nerve transfer

I. Principles of Tendon Transfer

- Injuries to the major nerves of the hand and upper extremity result in loss of function secondary to muscle paralysis, atrophy, and lack of sensibility.
- Depending on the chronicity and type of injury, nerve repair may not be an option. Tendon transfers are an option to reestablish motor function.
- Core principles of tendon transfers
  - Preoperative prevention of contracture: Full passive range of motion (ROM) of affected joints is required.
  - Preoperative tissue equilibrium: Scar tissue from previous trauma must be fully mature to provide a smooth bed for the transfer to function.
  - Adequate strength: Donor tendons must be from a muscle with appropriate strength.
  - Amplitude of motion: Excursion of the transferred tendon should match the required length of recipient tendon motion.
    - Flexors and extensors of the wrist have 30 mm of excursion.
    - Digital extensors have 50 mm of excursion.
    - Digital flexors have 70 mm of excursion.
  - Straight line of pull: Transferred tendons should be in as straight a line as possible from origin to insertion to reduce friction and optimize force transmission.
  - One function: A tendon should be transferred to execute a single action.
  - Synergism: Synergistic action of donor and recipient tendons should be considered (e.g., wrist flexion and finger extension are synergistic).
  - Expendable donor: Sacrifice of the donor tendon should not result in a loss of function, so there must be a separate muscle-tendon junction providing similar function.

II. Requirements for Tendon Transfers

- Passive ROM of all surrounding joints with supple web space skin.
- Radiographs to confirm no/minimal arthritic changes of surrounding joints.
- Ensure patient can be compliant with postoperative restrictions and occupational therapy protocols.

III. Tendon Transfers for Median Nerve Palsy

- Injuries are characterized as "high" or "low" depending on whether they occur above or below the anterior interosseous nerve (AIN) branch in the forearm.
- Low median nerve palsy
  - Thenar intrinsics including the opponens pollicis (OP), abductor pollicis brevis (AbPB), and the superficial head of the flexor pollicis brevis (FPB) are affected in addition to sensory innervation to the thumb/index/long/partial ring fingers.
  - Loss of thumb opposition is the primary motor deficit:
    - Opposition is multiplanar including abduction, pronation, and flexion.
    - Some opposition may be preserved by anatomically variable contributions from the ulnar nerve (Riche-Cannieu anastomosis).
    - The deep head of the FPB and the adductor pollicis (AdP) are innervated by the ulnar nerve, which may allow satisfactory compensation.
  - Tendon transfer to restore opposition (▶ Table 17.1):
    - Palmaris longus (PL) to AbPB/OP: PL is tunneled subcutaneously and attached to the AbPB/OP at the base of the thumb (a.k.a. Camitz transfer).
    - Extensor indicis proprius (EIP) to AbPB/OP: This will restore opposition even in the setting of a high median nerve palsy. EIP is transected on the dorsal aspect of the index finger just distal to the metacarpophalangeal (MCP) joint but proximal to the extensor hood, and freed proximal to the extensor retinaculum at the wrist. It is then routed subcutaneously in a volar ulnar direction over the flexor carpi ulnaris (FCU) to the AbPB/OP. Wrist is maintained in flexion for attachment.
    - Flexor digitorum sublimis (FDS) from the ring finger to AbPB/OP: The FDS to the ring finger is brought proximally and routed through a pulley created by a radial slip of FCU tendon (to create appropriate vector of pull) and then tunneled subcutaneously to the AbPB/OP.
    - Abductor digiti minimi (AbDM) to AbPB/OP (a.k.a. Huber transfer): AbDM is supplied by a neurovascular pedicle at the most dorsoradial aspect of its proximal

Table 17.1 Features of opponensplasty tendon transfer

Tendon transfer (Opponensplasty)	Features
PL to AbPB	Restore opposition
EIP to AbPB	Restore opposition
RF FDS to AbPB	Restore opposition
AbDM to AbPB	Restore opposition

Abbreviations: AbDM, abductor digiti minimi; AbPB, abductor pollicis brevis; EIP, extensor indicis proprius; FDS, flexor digitorum sublimis; PL, palmaris longus; RF-FDS, ring finger–flexor digitorum sublimis.

origin which must be protected during dissection and from being kinked as the tendon is tunneled to the APB. This option is usually used in children.

○ Postoperatively, a thumb spica splint is placed with the thumb in palmar abduction for 2 to 4 weeks and then protected ROM exercises are begun with occupational therapy.

- High median nerve palsy
  ○ The pronator teres (PT), flexor carpi radialis (FCR), FDS to all fingers, index and middle finger flexor digitorum profundus (FDP), flexor pollicis longus (FPL), and pronator quadratus (PQ) are affected, in addition to those affected in low median palsy.
  ○ The anterior interosseous nerve (AIN) off the main median nerve innervates some of the forearm musculature; therefore, AIN palsy mimics median nerve palsy, but spares the intrinsic muscles of the hand and has no associated sensory changes.
  ○ Loss of forearm pronation, thumb interphalangeal (IP) joint flexion, index finger flexion, and variable loss of long finger flexion are the main additional motor deficits. FCU provides wrist flexion in the absence of FCR.
  ○ Extensor carpi radialis longus (ECRL) to index finger (IF) FDP: The purpose of this transfer is to restore pinch. ECRL is identified in the distal forearm inserting at the base of the index finger metacarpal and transferred to the index finger FDP in the volar aspect of the forearm. A dorsal blocking splint is placed postoperatively to protect the repair, and active ROM is avoided for 4 weeks.
  ○ Brachioradialis (BR) to FPL to restore thumb IP joint flexion: The BR is identified at its insertion on the radial styloid, tunneled under the radial artery, and attached to the FPL deep to the FCR tendon. A thumb spica splint is placed postoperatively and active ROM is begun at 4 weeks (▶ Table 17.2).

IV. Tendon Transfers for Ulnar Nerve Palsy

- The ulnar nerve innervates the FCU, ring/small finger FDP muscles, hypothenar muscles, interossei muscles of the fingers, lumbricals for the ring/small finger, and the adductor pollicis.
- Clinical examination of low ulnar palsy shows a claw hand deformity from paralyzed intrinsics resulting in insufficient grasp patterns, small finger abduction, loss of strong key pinch, and ring/small finger IP flexion/MCP hyperextension resulting in loss of hand dexterity. In a more proximal ulnar palsy, the FDP to small and ring fingers are lost, and therefore the clawing of ring and small fingers may not occur.
  ○ Extensor digiti minimi (EDM), with radial nerve innervation, overpowers the paralyzed intrinsics to hold the small finger in abduction (Wartenberg's sign).

Table 17.2 Features of high median nerve injury tendon transfers

High median nerve injury tendon transfers	Features
ECRL to IF FDP	Restore pinch
BR to FPL	Restore thumb IP flexion

Abbreviations: BR, brachioradialis; ECRL, extensor carpi radialis longus; FPL, flexor pollicis longus; IF FDP, index finger flexor digitorum profundus; IP, interphalangeal.

- ○ Compensation of key pinch with thumb IP joint flexion, mediated by the FPL innervated by the median nerve, is known as Froment's sign. This is indicative of paralysis of the first dorsal interosseous and adductor pollicis.
- Transfers aid in avoiding claw hand position, restoring small finger abduction, and restoring ring and small finger distal IP joint function for grip strength.
  - ○ FDS middle finger transfer to correct claw deformity, dynamic intrinsicplasty: The FDS to the middle finger is transected under the A3 pulley after it has decussated into two limbs under the FDP. The two slips each serve as a donor tendon, tunneled to the radial lateral bands of the ring and small fingers at the level of the PIP joint. Transfers are tensioned with the wrist in neutral, MCP in 80 degrees of flexion, and the hand is placed in an intrinsic plus volar splint for 4 weeks.
  - ○ FDP side-to-side transfer to restore 4th/5th distal interphalangeal (DIP) flexion and grip strength (proximal ulnar nerve injury): The FDP tendons of the affected ring and small finger (SF) are sutured to the FDP of the middle finger and a dorsal blocking splint is placed postoperatively for 2 to 4 weeks.
  - ○ FDS lasso procedure, static intrinsicplasty: The FDS of the respective finger is identified at the level of the A3 pulley and transected at its distal insertion point after decussation. The FDS tendon is again identified just proximal to the A1 pulley and the transected slips are looped around the A1 pulley to be reattached to the proximal FDS tendon with the MCP in slight flexion. A dorsal blocking splint is applied for 3 weeks postoperatively.
- Transfers are also aimed at enhancing key pinch from the adductor pollicis, FPB, and first dorsal interossei.
  - ○ Extensor carpi radialis brevis (ECRB) with free tendon graft extension to AdP transfer to restore thumb adduction and key pinch: ECRB plus a 10 cm tendon graft is tunneled subcutaneously in the 3rd intermetacarpal space to use the long finger metacarpal as a pulley. It is then attached to the AdP tendon. The wrist is splinted with the thumb in neutral position for 4 weeks.
  - ○ Abductor pollicis longus (APL) transfer using tendon graft to restore index abduction: A radial slip of APL is taken at its insertion into the base of the first metacarpal. A tendon graft is then attached to the radial lateral band of the index finger MCP. The proximal end of the graft is tunneled to meet the radial slip of APL and tensioned to achieve radial abduction of the index finger. Repair is then immobilized with the wrist extended and padding between the index and middle fingers to maintain radial abduction for 4 weeks postoperatively (▶ Table 17.3).

V. Tendon Transfers for Radial Nerve Palsy

- Radial nerve/posterior interosseous nerve (PIN) injuries can result in deficits including loss of wrist and finger extension and lack of thumb extension/abduction. Management is more challenging if injury to the nerve is proximal to the elbow.
- Radial nerve splits into PIN (motor) and dorsal sensory after passing through the supinator muscle. Depending on the level of radial nerve/PIN injury, muscles that may be affected include the BR, ECRL, ECRB, supinator, extensor carpi ulnaris (ECU), EDM, APL, extensor pollicis brevis (EPB), and EIP. Each muscle must be tested to determine the intervention needed.
- The goal is to restore wrist and finger extension to facilitate pinch and grasp function, allowing for release of objects.

Table 17.3 Features of tendon transfer for ulnar palsy

Tendon transfer for ulnar palsy	Features
FDS MF to lateral bands of RF/SF	Dynamic intrinsicplasty
FDP side-to-side RF/SF to MF	Restore 4th/5th DIP flexion, enhance grip strength
FDS to itself over the A1 pulley	Static intrinsicplasty
ECRB to AdP (w/graft)	Restore thumb adduction, enhance key pinch
Radial slip APL to IF radial lateral band (w/graft)	Restore index finger abduction, enhance key pinch

Abbreviations: AdP, adductor pollicis; APL, abductor pollicis longus; DIP, distal interphalangeal; ECRB, extensor carpi radialis brevis; FDP, flexor digitorum profundus; FDS, flexor digitorum sublimis; IF, index finger; MF, middle finger; RF, ring finger; SF, small finger.

- PT to ECRB to restore wrist extension: The PT is passed over BR to be tied into ECRB. If radial nerve recovery is expected, the PT may be used to augment extension by tying it in side-to-side to ECRB as opposed to transecting ECRB at musculotendinous junction for formal coaptation. Transfer is tensioned with the wrist in 20 degrees of extension.
- FCR to extensor digitorum communis (EDC) transfer to restore finger extension: FCR is identified in the volar wrist, avoiding injury to the median nerve or radial artery, and transferred to the EDC in the dorsal forearm. The FCR is transferred into each individual slip of EDC and tensioned with the index finger in extension to reproduce the natural cascade.
- PL to extensor pollics longus (EPL) transfer to restore thumb IP extension: The PL is identified in the volar wrist and transferred to the EPL located over Lister's tubercle, with tension set with the thumb in a position of extension and abduction.
- FDS of the middle finger to EPL to restore thumb extension: If the PL is absent or it has been used for prior tendon graft, transfer of the FDS of the middle finger is an option. The FDS tendon is identified at the wrist and transferred subcutaneously over the dorsoradial border to the EPL (▶ Table 17.4).

VI. Nerve Transfers for Motor Preservation and Recovery

- Indications include patients with peripheral nerve injury who are expected to have a prolonged reinnervation time and at risk for loss of motor endplates, which are lost within 12 to 18 months.
- In the setting of pre-existing continuity of the nerve, such as a compression neuropathy, end-to-side transfer is recommended.
- A healing nerve grows at 1 to 2 mm per day (approximately 1 cm a month). Thus, nerve repair or grafting of proximal injuries results in poor outcomes from loss of motor endplates secondary to prolonged denervation.
- Preoperative electromyography (EMG) should be done to confirm viability of motor endplates in recipient musculature.

Table 17.4 Features of tendon transfer for radial nerve palsy

Tendon transfer for radial nerve palsy	Features
PT to ECRB	Restore wrist extension
FCR to EDC	Restore finger extension
PL to EPL	Restore thumb IP extension
FDS MF to EPL	Restore thumb IP extension

Abbreviations: ECRB, extensor carpi radialis brevis; EDC, extensor digitorum communis; EPL, extensor pollics longus; FCR, flexor carpi radialis; FDS MF, flexor digitorum sublimis middle finger; IP, interphalangeal; PL, palmaris longus; PT, pronator teres.

- Nerve stimulator can be helpful intraoperatively to help identify appropriate recipient nerve fascicles after acute transection (within about 72 hours). The donor nerve should be as close as possible to the target endplates to minimize reinnervation time.

VII. Nerve Transfers for Ulnar Neuropathy

- The most common nerve transfer for ulnar nerve injury is a distal AIN transfer to the motor branch of the ulnar nerve.
- The AIN is a motor branch of the median nerve arising 5 cm distal to the elbow and supplying the radial half of FDP, FPL, and PQ.
- Function of the AIN must be tested preoperatively by testing the FPL via thumb IP joint flexion, the FDP to the 1st or 2nd digits by testing DIP joint function, or the PQ by testing pronation with the elbow flexed so as to avoid pronation by the PT.
- At the wrist, the ulnar neurovascular bundle lies within Guyon's canal deep to the volar carpal ligament but superficial to the transverse carpal ligament.
- At the hook of the hamate, the ulnar nerve splits into a superficial sensory branch supplying the small and ring fingers, and deep motor branch supplying the intrinsics.
- Prior to this split, fascicles are arranged with motor fascicles ulnar and sensory fibers radial.
- More proximal in the forearm, the fascicles to the dorsal sensory branch are dorsal ulnar, the sensory fibers supplying the small/ring finger are dorsal radial, and motor fibers are central/volar (▶ Fig. 17.1).
- AIN is identified in the forearm just proximal to the PQ and transferred in a tension-free manner to the central motor fascicular group of the ulnar nerve. The hand is splinted in an intrinsic plus position for 2 to 3 weeks postoperatively.

VIII. Nerve Transfers for Median Neuropathy

- Transfer of the motor branch of the ECRB to the AIN, and the FCU branch of the ulnar nerve to the PT, in the case of proximal median nerve injury.
- Transfer of the FCU branch of the ulnar nerve to the AIN, and third lumbrical branch of ulnar nerve to the recurrent motor branch of the median nerve are also possibilities.
- Transfer of the dorsal sensory branch of the radial nerve to common digital nerves or median nerve is an option to restore sensation.

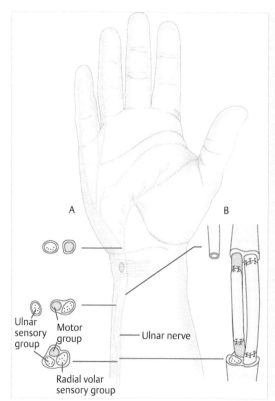

Fig. 17.1 Ulnar nerve fascicular topography. **A:** In the mid-forearm, there are three distinct fascicular groups: dorsal sensory branch, motor branch, and main sensory branch. **B:** Distal forearm nerve injuries can be more accurately reconstructed using one's knowledge of topography.

A   B

Ulnar sensory group
Motor group
Ulnar nerve
Radial volar sensory group

IX. Nerve Transfers for Radial Neuropathy

- Transfers from expendable median nerve FDS branches to the radial motor nerve branch of the ECRB, or FCR to the PIN have been described.
- The median motor nerve branches of the PT and the FCR transferred to radial motor nerve branches of the ECRB and the PIN have also been described.

Suggested Readings

Abrams RA, Ziets RJ, Lieber RL, Botte MJ. Anatomy of the radial nerve motor branches in the forearm. J Hand Surg Am. 1997; 22(2):232–237

Anderson GA. Ulnar nerve palsy. In Green D, et al, editors: Green's operative hand surgery, 2005, Elsevier, pp. 1161–1196

Beasley RW. Principles of tendon transfer. Orthop Clin North Am. 1970; 1(2):433–438

Dvali L, Mackinnon S. Nerve repair, grafting, and nerve transfers. Clin Plast Surg. 2003; 30(2):203–221

Goldner JL. Tendon transfers for irreparable peripheral nerve injuries of the upper extremity. Orthop Clin North Am. 1974; 5(2):343–375

Lee DH, Rodriguez JA, Jr. Tendon transfers for restoring hand intrinsic muscle function: a biomechanical study. J Hand Surg Am. 1999; 24(3):609–613

Lowe JB, III, Sen SK, Mackinnon SE. Current approach to radial nerve paralysis. Plast Reconstr Surg. 2002; 110 (4):1099–1113

Moussavi AA, Saied A, Karbalaeikhani A. Outcome of tendon transfer for radial nerve paralysis: Comparison of three methods. Indian J Orthop. 2011; 45(6):558–562

Novak CB, Mackinnon SE. Distal anterior interosseous nerve transfer to the deep motor branch of the ulnar nerve for reconstruction of high ulnar nerve injuries. J Reconstr Microsurg. 2002; 18(6):459–464

Omer GE. Tendon transfers for combined traumatic nerve palsies of the forearm and hand. J Hand Surg [Br]. 1992; 17(6):603–610

Omer GE, Jr. Reconstructive procedures for extremities with peripheral nerve defects. Clin Orthop Relat Res. 1982 (163):80–91

Ozkan T, Ozer K, Gülgönen A. Three tendon transfer methods in reconstruction of ulnar nerve palsy. J Hand Surg Am. 2003; 28(1):35–43

Rinker B. Nerve transfers in the upper extremity: a practical user's guide. Ann Plast Surg. 2015; 74(4) Suppl 4: S222–S228

Rinkinen JRMD, Giladi AMMD, Iorio ML. Outcomes Following Peripheral Nerve Transfers for Treatment of Non-Obstetric Brachial Plexus Upper-Extremity Neuropathy. JBJS Rev. 2018; 6(4):e1

Tung TH, Mackinnon SE. Nerve transfers: indications, techniques, and outcomes. J Hand Surg Am. 2010; 35 (2):332–341

18 Compression Neuropathies

Tyler Pidgeon, Samir Sabharwal, and Erica Taylor

Abstract

Peripheral nerve compression represents one of the most common reasons for presentation to hand surgery clinic. The most common peripheral nerve entrapment syndromes involve the median nerve, most frequently at the carpal tunnel, and the ulnar nerve, most commonly at the cubital tunnel. Although peripheral nerve anatomy generally lends to predictable patterns of symptomatology, some anomalies can exist. Thorough history and comprehensive, targeted physical examination are paramount to achieving an appropriate diagnosis. Given the time-dependent nature of nerve regeneration potential after mechanical decompression, it is important to implement appropriate treatment promptly.

Keywords: Compression neuropathy, carpal tunnel, cubital tunnel, median nerve, ulnar nerve, radial nerve

I. Peripheral Nerve Anatomy

- Neuron: Working unit of nervous system, composed of cell body along with axons and dendrites.
  - Axons: Larger processes with the function of conducting signals via action potentials:
    - Reside in the anterior horn in motor neurons, in the dorsal root ganglion in sensory neurons.
    - May be myelinated or unmyelinated.
  - Dendrites: Thinner processes with the function of receiving input from other nerves.
- Vasa nervorum are small arteries which supply peripheral nerves.
- Compression neuropathy, or nerve compression syndrome, is a condition caused by direct pressure on a peripheral nerve:
  - Direct compression induces local ischemia by reducing flow through the vasa nervorum.
  - Results in slowed action potentials, focal demyelination, axonal damage, and fibrosis.

II. Median Nerve Compression

A. Anatomic Course

- Arises from the medial and lateral cords of the brachial plexus, with input from C5 to T1.
- Gives off the anterior interosseous nerve (AIN) distal to the arch of the flexor digitorum superficialis (FDS).
  - AIN descends volar to the interosseous membrane between the radius and ulna, typically radial to the anterior interosseous artery.

- After innervating and passing dorsal to the pronator quadratus, the AIN terminates as sensory branches to the volar wrist capsule.
- Palmar cutaneous branch of the median nerve branches from the main nerve 5 to 7 cm proximal to the volar wrist crease:
  - Supplies sensation to the volar palm.
  - Runs between palmaris longus and flexor carpi radialis (FCR), passing volar to the transverse carpal ligament.
  - May run within the sheath of the FCR.
- Median nerve proper passes between FCR and FDS just proximal to the wrist, prior to entering the carpal tunnel.
- Recurrent motor branch travels radial to the median nerve through the carpal tunnel
  - Supplies thenar muscles.
- Distal to the carpal tunnel, the median nerve branches into radial and ulnar divisions
  - Radial division supplies sensation to the thumb and radial index finger via digital nerves.
  - Ulnar division supplies the ulnar index finger, middle finger, and radial ring finger via digital nerves.

B. Motor Innervation

- Pronator teres.
- Flexor carpi radialis.
- Palmaris longus.
- Flexor digitorum superficialis.
- Flexor digitorum profundus to index and long fingers (via anterior interosseous nerve).
- Flexor pollicis longus (via anterior interosseous nerve).
- Pronator quadratus (via anterior interosseous nerve).
- Flexor pollicis brevis (superficial head via recurrent motor branch).
- Abductor pollicis brevis (via recurrent motor branch).
- Opponens pollicis (via recurrent motor branch).
- First and second lumbricals (via digital nerves).

C. Sensory Innervation

- Articular branch to ulnohumeral joint.
- Volar palmar skin (via palmar cutaneous nerve).
- Volar thumb, index finger, middle finger, and radial half of ring finger.

D. Potential Compression Points

- Pectoralis minor.
- Anomalous axillary vascular structures.
- Supracondylar process.
  - Projects anteromedially from the anterior humeral shaft, approximately 3 to 5 cm proximal to the medial epicondyle, best seen on oblique radiographs of the humerus.
  - Only present in about 1% of individuals.

- Connected to the medial epicondyle via ligament of Struthers:
    - The median nerve may be compressed as it passes underneath the ligament of Struthers, between the supracondylar process and medial epicondyle.
- Gantzer's muscle
    - Anomalous muscle, present in 45% of limbs.
    - Arises from the medial condyle of the humerus, inserts into the flexor pollicis longus.
- Lacertus fibrosis.
- Pronator teres.
- Arch of the flexor digitorum superficialis.
- Palmaris profundus
    - Anomalous muscle that originates proximal to the flexor pollicis longus from the radius, inserts onto the transverse carpal ligament.
- Flexor capri radialis brevis
    - Anomalous muscle that originates near the proximal origin of the flexor pollicis longus from the radius, inserts onto the flexor carpi radialis.
- Ulnar collateral artery.
- Aberrant branches of radial artery to anterior interosseous nerve.
- Carpal tunnel
    - Fibro-osseous tunnel in the volar wrist; finger and thumb flexors travel with the median nerve on their way to the hand.
    - Borders include the transverse carpal ligament volarly, the carpal bones dorsally, the hook of the hamate and triquetrum ulnarly, and the scaphoid tubercle and trapezium radially.
    - Anatomic variants such as a transligamentous recurrent motor branch may put the nerve at risk during surgical release (▸ Fig. 18.1).

E. Carpal Tunnel Syndrome

1. Diagnosis

- Symptoms include numbness and paresthesias in the sensory distribution of the median nerve distal to the wrist, weakness of the thenar musculature, and nocturnal awakening.
- Six-Item Carpal Tunnel Syndrome (CTS-6) scale aids diagnosis and predicts response to surgical release:
    - Symptoms in the median nerve distribution.
    - Nocturnal numbness.
    - Thenar atrophy or weakness.
    - Positive Phalen's test.
    - Positive Tinel's sign.
    - Loss of two-point discrimination.
- Ultrasound and electrodiagnostic testing may confirm diagnosis.

2. Management

- Nonoperative
    - Immobilization with night-time splinting.
    - Nonsteroidal anti-inflammatory drugs (NSAIDs).
    - Corticosteroid injection.

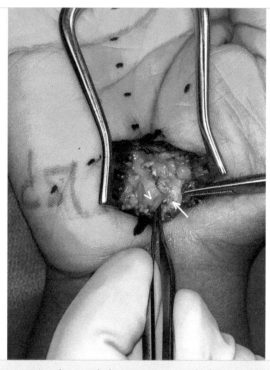

Fig. 18.1 This intraoperative photograph demonstrates a standard "mini-open" approach to release of the carpal tunnel. In this patient, a rare transligamentous recurrent motor branch of the median nerve was encountered. The arrow without a tail demonstrates the recurrent motor branch which is being lifted by forceps. The arrow with a tail points at the pathway of the recurrent motor branch through the transverse carpal ligament to the thenar muscles. This pathway is also being demonstrated by a hemostat.

- Surgical decompression
  - Open carpal tunnel release.
  - Endoscopic carpal tunnel release (**Video 18.1**).

III. Ulnar Nerve Compression

A. Anatomic Course

- Formed from the medial cord of the brachial plexus, made up of fibers from C8 to T1.
- Passes posterior to the pectoralis major and medial to the brachial artery as it enters the anterior compartment of the arm; crosses the medial intermuscular septum to enter the posterior compartment approximately 8 cm proximal to the medial epicondyle of the humerus.
- Travels posterior to the insertion of the medial intermuscular septum onto the medial humeral epicondyle, to enter the cubital tunnel:
  - Covered by Osborne's ligament.

o Exits the cubital tunnel to enter the forearm between the two heads of the flexor carpi ulnaris.
- Prior to entering Guyon's canal, gives off dorsal sensory branch.

B. Motor Innervation

- Flexor carpi ulnaris.
- Flexor digitorum profundus to ring and small fingers.
- Abductor digiti minimi.
- Flexor digiti minimi.
- Opponens digiti minimi.
- Interossei.
- Third and fourth lumbricals.
- Flexor pollicis brevis (deep head).
- Adductor pollicis.

C. Sensory Innervation

- Articular branch to ulnohumeral joint.
- Dorsal ulnar hand, small finger, and ring finger (via dorsal sensory branch of the ulnar nerve).
- Volar small finger and ulnar ring finger.

D. Potential Compression Points

- First rib.
- Arcade of Struthers
  o Variably found in 20 to 70% of individuals.
  o Thick fascial band connecting the medial head of the triceps to the medial intermuscular septum, approximately 4 to 10 cm proximal to the medial epicondyle.
- Medial head of the triceps.
- Cubital tunnel
  o Fibro-osseous tunnel, made up of inferior portion of medial epicondyle superolaterally and Osborne's ligament inferomedially.
  o Represents the most common compression point of the ulnar nerve.
  o The anconeus epitrochlearis, an anomalous muscle that spans the medial epicondyle to the medial border of the olecranon, may join the ulnar nerve in the cubital tunnel and further reduce the space available (▶ Fig. 18.2).
    – Found in 1 to 30% of individuals.
- Flexor carpi ulnaris.
- Guyon's canal
  o Nerve enters the approximately 4.5 cm canal with ulnar artery, volar to transverse carpal ligament.
  o Bordered by FCU, pisiform, and abductor digiti minimi (ADM) ulnarly, transverse carpal ligament and hook of the hamate radially, palmaris brevis palmarly, and pisohamate and pisometacarpal ligaments dorsally.
  o Bifurcates into sensory and motor branches within canal.

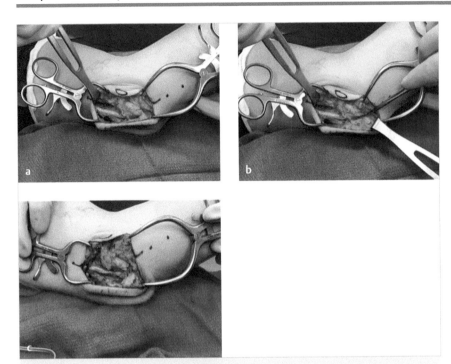

Fig. 18.2 (a–c) Intraoperative image of an accessory muscle, anconeus epitrochlearis, serving as a point of entrapment for the ulnar nerve along the medial elbow.

- Motor branch runs deep, wraps around hook of the hamate and innervates adductor digiti minimi and flexor digiti minimi as it passes in between; follows deep palmar arch radially.
- Sensory branch runs superficial, exits canal at distal margin of hypothenar muscles; continues distally to form digital nerves.
    ○ Nerve may be compressed by native structures of the canal, or by space-occupying lesions, such as ganglion cyst or ulnar artery aneurysm.

E. Cubital Tunnel Syndrome

1. Diagnosis

- Second most common upper extremity nerve compression pathology, after carpal tunnel syndrome.
- Symptoms: Focal medial elbow pain; paresthesias/dysthesias radiating along the volar ulnar forearm; numbness of the small finger and ulnar half of the ring finger; clumsiness of the hand secondary to intrinsic weakness.
    ○ Those with intermittent, positional symptoms have a more predictable outcome than those with constant numbness.
- Examination findings: Disturbed moving touch; reduced vibratory sensation; reduced two-point discrimination over the small finger and ulnar side of the ring finger; intrinsic muscle wasting.

- Wartenberg's sign: Ulnar deviation of the small finger and weakness of small finger adduction due to intrinsic muscle paralysis.
- Froment's sign: Severely diminished key pinch strength secondary to reduced adductor pollicis function, causing patients to pinch via thumb interphalangeal (IP) joint flexion (flexor pollicis longus innervated by the anterior interosseous nerve).
- Provocative maneuvers: Combined elbow flexion-pressure test; Tinel's sign at the elbow.
- Ultrasound and electrodiagnostic testing may confirm diagnosis.

2. Management

- Nonoperative
  - Activity modification, avoiding prolonged elbow flexion.
  - NSAIDs.
  - Night-time elbow extension splinting.
- Operative
  - Simple decompression
    - Open approach.
    - Endoscopic approach.
  - Open decompression with transposition—favored in those with nerve subluxation or failed simple decompression
    - Subcutaneous transposition.
    - Intramuscular transposition.
    - Submuscular transposition.
  - Medial epicondylectomy.
  - Superior results in younger patients and those treated within 6 months of symptom onset.
  - Optimal treatment option remains controversial.

IV. Radial Nerve Compression

A. Anatomic Course

- Formed from posterior cord of brachial plexus, with input from C5 to T1.
- Passes through triangular interval, descends in posterior compartment with profunda brachii artery.
- Pierces lateral intermuscular septum in distal third of humerus, into anterior compartment.
- After passing lateral epicondyle into forearm, divides into superficial branch (▶ Fig. 18.3) and posterior interosseous nerve (PIN):
  - Superficial branch of the radial nerve (SBRN) provides sensation to the dorsal radial wrist and hand.
  - PIN passes deep to the arcade of Frohse through the deep and superficial heads of the supinator; gives off branches to wrist and finger extensors as it descends past; then travels deep to the fourth dorsal compartment adjacent to the posterior interosseous artery, innervating the dorsal wrist capsule.

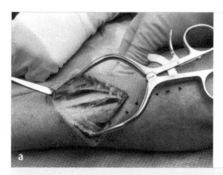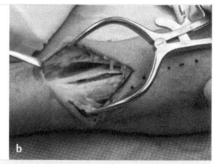

Fig. 18.3 (a, b) The superficial branch of the radial nerve at its proximal origin.

B. Motor Innervation

- Triceps.
- Brachialis (lateral).
- Anconeus.
- Brachioradialis.
- Extensor carpi radialis longus.
- Extensor carpi radialis brevis.
- Extensor carpi ulnaris (via posterior interosseous nerve).
- Extensor digitorum communis (via posterior interosseous nerve).
- Extensor digiti minimi (via posterior interosseous nerve).
- Abductor pollicis longus (via posterior interosseous nerve).
- Extensor pollicis longus (via posterior interosseous nerve).
- Extensor pollicis brevis (via posterior interosseous nerve).
- Extensor indicis proprius (via posterior interosseous nerve).

C. Sensory Innervation

- Posterior lateral arm (via posterior brachial sensory nerve).
- Ulnohumeral joint.
- Dorsal wrist/hand (via superfical branch of the radial nerve).
- Dorsal wrist joint (via posterior interosseous nerve).

D. Potential Compression Points

- Anomalous axillary vascular structures.
- Anomalous axillary musculature.
- Lateral head of the triceps.
- Lateral intermuscular septum.
- Radiocapitellar joint capsule.
- Recurrent radial artery/leash of Henry.
- Tendinous margin of the extensor carpi radialis brevis.
- Supinator/arcade of Frohse
  - Fascial band approximately 5 cm distal to the lateral epicondyle, representing the leading edge of the supinator.

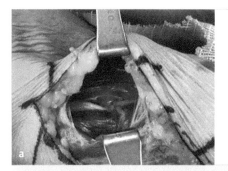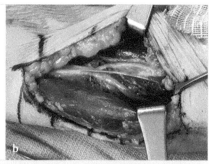

Fig. 18.4 (a, b) Intraoperative imaging of the radial tunnel during surgical decompression.

- Common compression point for the posterior interosseous branch of the radial nerve, as it passes deep to the supinator descending distally in the forearm.
- Nerve may also be compressed at the distal aspect of the supinator.
- Brachioradialis/extensor carpi radialis longus (SBRN).
  - Wartenberg's syndrome: Compression of the SBRN as it pierces through the fascia of the brachioradialis and extensor carpi radialis longus.

1. Diagnosis

- Patients may present with deep, aching proximal forearm pain or a sensation of heaviness.
- Light palpation over the proximal margin of the supinator may reproduce symptoms.
- Resisted forearm supination with wrist extension or resisted long finger extension has been proposed as provocative maneuvers.
- Nerve conduction study (NCS)/electromyography (EMG) is unreliable in detecting radial nerve compression.

2. Management

- Nonoperative—should be tried for 3 months
  - Activity modification—avoid elbow extension with forearm pronation and wrist flexion, as this exacerbates compression of the radial nerve.
  - NSAIDs.
  - Splinting and therapy.
- Operative management
  - Decompression of PIN via open release of supinator and arcade of Frohse (▶ Fig. 18.4).

Suggested Readings

Boone S, Gelberman RH, Calfee RP. The management of cubital tunnel syndrome. J Hand Surg Am. 2015; 40 (9):1897–1904, quiz 1904

Bickel KD. Carpal tunnel syndrome. J Hand Surg Am. 2010; 35(1):147–152

Dang AC, Rodner CM. Unusual compression neuropathies of the forearm, part I: radial nerve. J Hand Surg Am. 2009; 34(10):1906–1914

Szabo RM, Gelberman RH. The pathophysiology of nerve entrapment syndromes. J Hand Surg Am. 1987; 12(5 Pt 2):880–884

19 Soft Tissue Reconstruction: Hand and Upper Extremity

Manas Nigam and Ryan Katz

Abstract

Soft tissue injuries to the arm, and or fingers must be addressed in a timely fashion with a goal toward restoring the injured part with the highest quality tissue. Failure to do so will often result in a stiff joint, unstable scar, and/or dysfunction of the extremity. Thus, the principle of "replace like with like" is often invoked. This chapter has been constructed to educate and illustrate the reconstructive options available to the surgeon who is treating soft tissue injuries of the hand and upper extremity.

Keywords: Open wound, local flap, regional flap, pedicled flap, free flap, hand, arm, finger

I. Introduction

- Upper extremity injury can involve bone, tendon, nerve, vessels, soft tissue, and skin.
  - The reconstruction should ideally "replace like with like."
  - Soft tissue coverage options should consider donor site morbidity.
  - Optimize wound healing and functional outcomes with the following principles:
    - Catalog all injured structures requiring repair.
    - Debride back to healthy tissues (may require multiple debridements).
    - Delay bone, tendon, and nerve repair/reconstruction until the time of definitive soft tissue coverage.
    - Provide stable bone fixation and strong tendon repairs to allow for early motion.
    - Resurface wounds with healthy soft tissue coverage that is supple and minimizes dead space.
- Delay reconstruction in the face of life-threating injuries; temporary coverage with allograft or xenograft or managing open wounds with a negative pressure dressing can allow for time between injury and formal reconstruction.
- A multidisciplinary team approach will allow comprehensive care: Upper extremity surgeon, physical and occupational therapy, and psychologist or psychiatrist.
- Sometimes amputation is functionally the best treatment:
  - If the expected result is a stiff or insensate part.
  - If the injured part impairs the global function of the arm or hand.
  - If the part is grossly contaminated, has segmental injuries, and/or cannot be salvaged.
- Evaluate patient's comorbid conditions and overall health:
  - History of cardiac disease, pulmonary disease, bleeding, or thrombophilic disorder can affect reconstruction options.
  - Occupation matters: A manual laborer requiring strength may benefit from a different reconstruction than a musician requiring dexterity.
- For severe crushing, mangling injury, defer final reconstruction for at least 24 to 48 hours after the injury.
  - To allow for complete demarcation of tissues.

○ To allow for adequate debridement.
○ Ischemia and inadequate resuscitation can extend the zone of tissue necrosis:
  – Muscle, skin, and then bone have increasing tolerances to ischemia—muscle can survive for 4 to 6 hours.
• Whenever possible, select the soft tissue reconstruction that can deliver the prerequisites of a dexterous extremity:
  ○ Supple skin.
  ○ Sensation.
  ○ Muscle tendon glide/continuity.
  ○ Posture and position allowing interaction with the environment, hygiene, and avoidance of trauma.
• Address postoperative access to therapy, clinic visits, medical needs, and psychologic counseling prior to discharge.

II. Finger

A. Anatomic Considerations

• Palmar glabrous skin
  ○ Resistant to shear forces due to high coefficient of static friction and papillary ridges (forming individual characteristic fingerprints).
  ○ Sensation with discrimination (narrow static and two-point discrimination).
• Dorsal nonglabrous skin
  ○ Thin, soft, and mobile.
  ○ Often hair bearing in males.
  ○ Sensation (less discrimination than palmar skin).

B. Distal Coverage

• Goal: Sensate glabrous skin where missing or nail elements where missing.
• Secondary intention (small fingertip defects):
  ○ Wounds of up to 2 cm.
  ○ Injuries without exposed bone, nerve, or tendon can be allowed to heal secondarily.
  ○ Even small wounds of the distal finger with healthy appearing exposed bone can often heal by secondary intention.
  ○ Daily dressing changes:
    – Keep the wound clean with daily washes or soaks.
    – Keep the wound moist with an ointment.
  ○ The result is often one of good sensation, and contour with no donor site morbidity.
  ○ Motion throughout the healing process can help minimize stiffness.
  ○ Wounds larger than 2 to 3 cm may benefit from surgical intervention.
• Primary closure.
• Cap graft:
  ○ In a distal fingertip amputation, for children less than 10 years of age, the amputated part may be sutured to the tip as a composite graft, after defatting as a "cap graft".[1,2]
  ○ Graft take is 7%, with a majority of patients experiencing partial graft failure.
  ○ Reoperation rates with cap or composite grafts is 10%.[3]

1. Local Flaps

- Homodigital flap (▶ Fig. 19.1):
  - Neurovascular island flap based on radial or ulnar digital artery.
  - Can cover tip, pulp, and dorsal wounds.
  - Can be used based on anterograde or retrograde blood supply:
    - Anterograde homodigital island flap is immediately sensate.[4]
    - Retrograde homodigital island flap is not immediately sensate.
  - Given the immediate sensation, an anterograde homodigital island flap is often preferred:
    - A proximal interphalangeal (PIP) flexion contracture is a commonly cited risk of the flap (but not often a clinical finding or, when present, of clinical significance).
  - If raised as a retrograde flap, the nerve may either be included or excluded from the flap:
    - If included, the nerve has to be coapted to the contralateral distal nerve for the prospect of sensation.
    - Excluding the nerve, although possible, could compromise flap venous drainage.
  - The anterograde flap is designed by making a template of the wound and transposing the template directly above the distal aspect of the radial or ulnar digital artery (surgeon's preference).
    - Harvesting the flap from the ulnar aspect of the digit usually results in less noticeable scar.
  - The flap can be slightly less than the size of the wound.
  - The flap is raised by preserving all soft tissue attachments between the skin and the neurovascular bundle (like a balloon on a string).
  - Great care is taken to not over-dissect the pedicle:
    - The venous drainage of the flap is likely the periadventitial tissues which should be protected by avoiding pedicle skeletonization.
    - The nerve and artery should be kept together throughout the dissection.
  - The flap donor site can be managed with a skin graft.
  - The hand is splinted with the digits in slight flexion for 3 weeks after which time, no splinting is required.
    - Range of motion exercises are allowed during this period of protection.
- Atasoy or volar V-Y advancement flap
  - Pedicled flaps often used for distal transverse or dorsal oblique fingertip defects

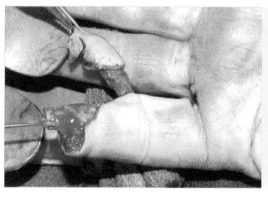

Fig. 19.1 Anterograde homodigital island flap.

- Atasoy (V-Y) should be designed such that the base of the "V" should not cross the distal interphalangeal (DIP) flexion crease:[5]
    - Cuts should be made only to release dermal attachments.
    - Cuts should not be made full thickness as this will compromise the blood supply of the flap.
  - These flaps are contraindicated for defects with more volar than dorsal skin loss.
  - Deep fibrous septa that anchor the glabrous skin to the underlying phalanx can be released with an elevator or knife but the superficial subcutaneous tissue should be retained.
  - Up to 1 cm advancement is theoretically achievable.
  - Functional and cosmetic results are excellent with this flap.
  - There exists a risk of cold intolerance and dysesthesia with this method.[6]
- Kutler or lateral V-Y advancement flap
  - Indicated for transverse and lateral oblique fingertip defects.
  - Flap uses lateral V-Y advancements lateral to the wound.
  - Elevated similar to the volar V-Y advancement flap in the plane of the neurovascular bundle above the flexor tendon sheath.
  - Kutler flaps should be designed to preserve the flap's blood supply from each digital artery:
    - The dorsal cut can be full thickness to periosteum.
    - The volar cut should be deep enough to release dermal attachments but should not be made full thickness.
    - Full-thickness volar cuts would transect the digital arterial blood supply to the digit.
  - Limited flap mobility allows minimal coverage.
  - There exists a risk of cold intolerance and dysesthesia.[7]
- Adipofascial turnover flap (▶ Fig. 19.2)
  - Pedicled homodigital flap often used when other methods are unavailable.
  - The skin is incised and elevated off the underlying fat.
  - A distal "pedicle" of fat is marked and protected from dissection.
  - The adipofascial tissue is then incised as a rectangular flap and elevated in a proximal to distal fashion.
  - The flap is brought distally, flipping it over the pedicle, and sutured in place to cover the defect.
  - The adipofascial tissue can then be skin grafted.

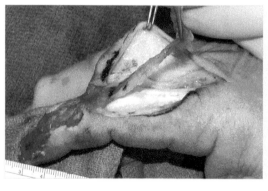

Fig. 19.2 Adipofascial turnover flap.

C. Proximal Coverage

- Goal: Coverage of vital structures, preservation of function (by providing gliding planes and sensate tissue), and restoration of form.
- Small wounds can be allowed to heal via secondary intention.
- Small wounds amenable to primary closure can be closed after a thorough washout.
- Larger wounds that cannot be closed primarily or would take excessive time to heal secondarily should be managed with a flap.

1. Cross Finger Flap

- Dorsal skin used as a pedicle flap to resurface volar defects (▶ Fig. 19.3):
  - The flap is insensate.
  - The flap brings nonglabrous skin to a previously glabrous area.
  - The flap is an example of an interpolated flap.
- The flap is outlined on an adjacent finger keeping the pedicle radial for flaps destined to be transferred radial or ulnar for flaps destined to be transferred ulnar.
- The skin is elevated off the extensor tendon taking care to preserve the paratenon (to facilitate skin graft take at the donor site).
- The flap is inset into the defect and the fingers are effectively (and purposefully) syndactylized.
- The flap is often divided at 3 weeks.
- Stiffness is an often-cited risk factor especially in patients with advanced age (> 50 years), osteoarthritis, or both.

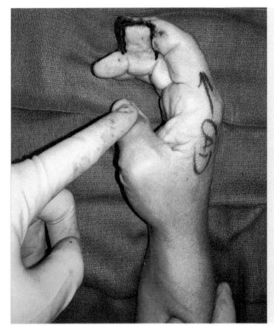

Fig. 19.3 Cross finger flap.

2. Reverse Cross Finger Flap

- Dorsal adipofascial tissue used to resurface dorsal wounds:
  - The flap is insensate.
  - The flap does not have skin and, as such, requires a skin graft.
- The flap is raised from an adjacent finger with an incision made on the side of the finger toward the defect (the incision should be ulnar for a defect on an ulnar digit and radial for a defect on a radial digit).
- A skin flap is then elevated in the immediate sub-dermal plane taking care to protect the adipofascial tissue beneath.
- The adipofascial tissue is raised as a pedicle flap by raising it off the extensor tendon.
  - The paratenon needs not be protected here as the tendon will be covered by the overlying skin upon closure.
- The flap is flipped over on itself and inset into the defect effectively (and purposefully) syndactylizing the digit.
- A split or full-thickness skin graft is applied to the flap.
- The elevated skin on the donor finger is closed over the extensor tendon taking care not to kink or apply pressure to the adipofascial flap pedicle.
- The flap is divided at 3 weeks.
- Motion is initiated once the skin graft appears adherent.
- Mobilization is immediate.

3. Skin Graft

- Considered as a means of reconstruction when extent of defect is limited to skin (▶ Fig. 19.4).
- Skin graft directly on nerve or bone is poorly tolerated and is often unstable (prone to breakdown).
- Full- or split-thickness skin graft can cover a well-vascularized bed.
  - Fascia, muscle, peritenon, and periosteum can all support a skin graft.
- Harvest split-thickness skin graft of 0.008 to 0.015 inch with a knife or dermatome.
- Split-thickness skin grafts can be harvested from anywhere on the body:
  - Common donor sites are the thigh, abdomen, and back.
  - Multiple grafts can be taken from the same donor site, limited only by the thickness of the dermis.
  - Meshed split grafts have the greatest amount of initial surface coverage.
  - Meshed split grafts have the greatest amount of delayed contraction and scarring.
- Full-thickness skin grafts incorporate the entire dermal layer and are usually hand harvested with a knife.

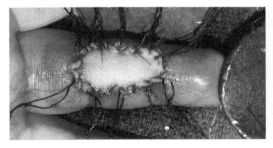

Fig. 19.4 Examples of skin graft.

- Full-thickness skin graft donor sites are more limited than split:
  - Common donor sites are hypothenar eminence (to resurface glabrous skin), volar forearm or medial upper arm (for hairless nonglabrous skin), and groin (for large area needing coverage).
  - Full-thickness grafts have the greatest amount of primary contraction and the least amount of initial surface coverage.
  - Full-thickness grafts have the least amount of secondary contraction.
  - Full-thickness grafts have the full dermis including dermal appendages and therefore, once healed, will be supple, elastic, can be hair bearing, and will have normal skin properties.
- Full-thickness grafts taken from antecubital fossa or wrist crease may result in undesirable scars.
  - A transverse scar at the wrist crease may carry the stigma of a prior suicide attempt.
- Be wary of color mismatches
  - Split grafts often lose pigment and can appear pink.
  - Dark grafts on the palm are often visible and can draw unwanted attention.
- Skin graft failure is often the result of either a poor graft bed, fluid accumulation under the graft, or shear forces below the graft.
  - Preparation of wound bed by debridement of devitalized tissues is paramount.
  - Meshing the graft (or making small slits within it) will limit fluid accumulation by allowing egress.
    - The average meshing ratio is 1:1.5; a ratio of 1:2 will allow for greater surface coverage but can be more challenging to work with.
  - Splinting for at least 1 week after grafting will minimize motion shear forces and motion under the graft.
- Using negative pressure wound therapy limits fluid accumulation under the graft and minimizes motion and shear forces.

4. Integra (Integra, Integra LifeSciences Co., Plainsboro, NJ)

- Bovine collagen and shark chondroitin-6-sulfate covered by a silicone layer (▶ Fig. 19.5).

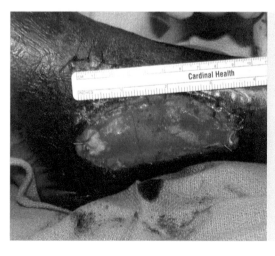

Fig. 19.5 Example of Integra.

- Acellular dermal substitute:
  - Because it is acellular, it will not be susceptible to necrosis and can therefore be placed on wound beds lacking well-vascularized surfaces.
  - Revascularizes from the periphery toward the center.
  - Requires a clean (uncontaminated and not infected) wound bed.
- The scaffold allows for ingrowth of cells and vessels into the matrix.
- Is often used with negative pressure wound therapy.
- Can be used in a layered fashion to build up thickness.
- Requires a thin split-thickness skin graft once the acellular matrix has revascularized.

III. Thumb

- Goals of reconstruction: Length, motion, sensibility, supple first web space, and appropriate aesthetic.
  - Loss of the thumb at or distal to the interphalangeal (IP) joint is usually well tolerated and may not require reconstruction. Amputation at this level is considered "compensated."
  - Amputation of the thumb proximal to the IP joint is usually not well tolerated and may benefit from reconstruction. Amputation at this level is considered "uncompensated."
  - Pulp loss would benefit from resurfacing with stable skin.
  - Preservation of carpometacarpal (CMC) joint motion is key. A stiff IP and/or MCP joint is usually well tolerated.

A. First Dorsal Metacarpal Artery (FDMA) Flap

- The FDMA can be used to resurface dorsal or volar thumb defects (▶ Fig. 19.6).
- Can provide dorsoradial sensory nerve sensation to volar pulp.
- The flap is harvested from the dorsal aspect of the index finger proximal phalanx:
  - The skin is raised in a full-thickness fashion (preserving paratenon on the extensor tendon to allow for skin grafting of the donor defect).
  - The flap is raised with the fascia of the first dorsal interosseous (FDI) muscle.
  - The flap pedicle is included with the fascia of the FDI and is purposefully not skeletonized (overdissection could injure the pedicle).

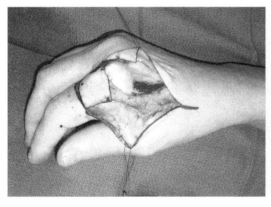

Fig. 19.6 First dorsal metacarpal artery flap.

- The flap is mobilized only as much as needed to transfer it to the thumb.
  - The flap can be tunneled under the skin overlying the ulnar aspect of the thumb as this skin is usually quite pliable.
- The size of the flap should be designed slightly larger than the defect.
- Before transposition flap viability is tested by releasing the tourniquet.
- The flap is then transposed through a tunnel to cover the thumb defect.
- The wound can be incised proximally or the tunnel can be completely released if there is any concern for pressure on the pedicle.
- The donor site is resurfaced with a full-thickness skin graft:
  - The skin graft is "piecrusted" and secured to the index finger donor site wound bed with a "bolster dressing" of Vaseline gauze, cotton, and mineral oil.
  - The bolster dressing minimizes fluid collection under the graft.
  - Splinting the index finger in extension minimizes shear forces under the graft.
  - Index (donor) finger motion can begin at 1 week once the bolster dressing has been removed.
- Thumb motion can begin usually within 3 weeks once the flap has incorporated into the surrounding soft tissues.

B. Moberg Flap

- The Moberg flap is a bipedicled neurovascular island flap mobilized on the radial and ulnar neurovascular bundles of the thumb (▶ Fig. 19.7).
  - It is an example of an anterograde homodigital island flap.
  - Often used for volar soft tissue defects of the thumb pulp.
- This flap provides an excellent sensory outcome without the need for cortical reorientation.
- The flap can be advanced to cover up to 2 cm defects.
- Meets the ideal of "replacing like with like" tissue.
- Can be raised without risk to the dorsal skin given the thumb's unique dorsal vasculature.
- The flap is raised off the underlying fibro-osseous sheath of the flexor pollicis:
  - Optimal advancement can be gained by making a back-cut at the level of the MP joint flexion crease and truly islandizing the flap on the radial and ulnar neurovascular bundles.
  - A back-cut is not necessary for flaps that require minimal distal advancement.
  - The IP joint can be flexed to facilitate distal coverage:
    - If the IP joint is flexed, motion should begin as soon as the flap appears to be incorporating into the surrounding soft tissues (1–3 weeks).
    - Flexion of the IP joint usually does not result in stiffness at this level.

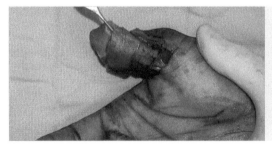

Fig. 19.7 Moberg flap.

- Postoperatively, a dorsal blocking thumb spica splint is applied to prevent full extension and undue tension on the flap pedicle.
- Splinting can be discontinued at 3 weeks.

C. Toe Pulp Flap (Free Tissue)

- This flap from the great toe achieves the ideal of replacing "like with like" tissue (▶ Fig. 19.8).
  - Provides sensate glabrous skin and can achieve excellent sensory and aesthetic outcomes.
- The flap is harvested from the great toe, is based off the first dorsal metatarsal artery, and includes one or both digital nerves.
- The flap nerve(s) are coapted to the thumb digital nerves in a tension-free manner:
  - The nerve coaptation should be performed as distally as possible to minimize the distance from proximal nerve to distal sensory end-organ.
- The flap requires microsurgical expertise to perform the arterial and venous anastomoses as well as the nerve coaptations.
- The flap donor site (great toe) is usually closed with a skin graft.
- Weight bearing on the foot should be minimized for 3 weeks to limit postoperative edema.
- Thumb range of motion can begin once the flap incorporates into the surrounding soft tissues (approximately 3 weeks).

IV. Hand

- Goals of reconstruction: Cover vital structures, including blood vessels, bone, nerves, and/or tendons.

A. Dorsal Hand

1. Reverse Radial Forearm Flap

- Prior to harvest, must confirm adequate collateral flow to the hand via the ulnar artery.
  - An Allen's test can demonstrate adequacy of collateral flow.

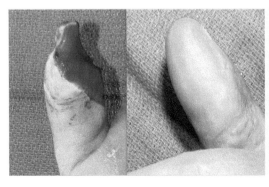

Fig. 19.8 Free toe pulp flap.

- If distal capillary refill is delayed or poor while the examiner is holding the radial artery occluded during an Allen's test, the radial artery should not be harvested.
- This flap brings thin supple soft tissue from the proximal forearm to the dorsal hand (or first web space).
- The "reverse" nature of the flap speaks to the retrograde flow from the radial artery and draining venae comitans:
  - The veins drain in a distal to proximal fashion through multiple "step-ladder" bridging connections between the venae.
- The flap is harvested in a full-thickness fashion, with fascia, off the flexor carpi radialis (FCR) and brachioradialis (BR).
  - The radial artery and a thin septum between the FCR and BR are protected and harvested with the flap.
  - The plane of dissection is subfascial and below the radial artery.
  - The tourniquet may be released and a noncrushing clamp may be applied to the distal radial artery to confirm adequate circulation to the hand prior to division of the proximal radial artery.
- The pivot point is typically the radial artery at the level of the radial styloid.
- The cephalic vein can be taken with the flap to provide for additional venous outflow (if needed) with microvascular anastomosis.
- Branches of the lateral antebrachial cutaneous nerve can be harvested with the flap and anastomosed to recipient nerves for potential flap sensation.
- The donor site is managed with either a split- or full-thickness skin graft.

2. Posterior Interosseous Artery (PIA) Flap

- This fasciocutaneous island flap is based on retrograde flow through the PIA (▶ Fig. 19.9).
- The artery runs in the interval between the extensor carpi ulnaris (ECU) and extensor digiti quinti (EDQ) and travels in a line from the lateral epicondyle toward the distal radioulnar joint (DRUJ):
  - The artery has an anastomosis with the anterior interosseous artery approximately 2 cm proximal to the DRUJ.
  - This anastomosis is thus the pivot point for this flap.
- The flap is raised in a full-thickness fashion, preserving the septum between the ECU and EDQ through which the perforators run.
- The wrist can be extended to increase the relative reach of the flap.
- The flap is often used to resurface the first web space and dorsal hand.

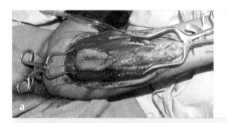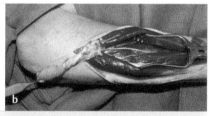

Fig. 19.9 Posterior interosseous artery (PIA) flap (anterograde and retrograde).

- Although donor site defects of 3 to 4 cm may be closed, larger ones should receive a skin graft.

3. Groin Flap: Pedicled and Free

- The groin flap provides a large surface area of thin and pliable skin coverage of the hand or fingers (▶ Fig. 19.10).
- The superficial circumflex iliac artery (SCIA), a branch of the superficial femoral artery, supplies the flap.
- The SCIA can be located with a doppler running parallel to and below the inguinal ligament.
- The flap can be raised either as a pedicled or free flap:
  - The flap is often raised in a lateral to medial fashion.
  - The dissection proceeds to the sartorius fascia which can be incised and raised with the flap (for a margin of safety) or left behind if a suprafascial perforator is visualized within the flap.
  - The descending branch of the lateral femoral circumflex nerve should be identified and protected.
  - If pedicled, the base can be tubularized for hygiene.
  - If free, consider harvesting extra veins to be utilized as needed to augment venous outflow if congestion is noted ("supercharging").
  - The donor site, which can almost always be closed primarily, should be closed over a drain to minimize seromas.
  - Tension on the closure can be relieved by temporarily flexing the hip.
- Pedicled flaps should be divided at 3 weeks (by this time, the flap is no longer dependent on its axial blood supply):
  - Pedicled flaps should be considered for patients who are unable to tolerate a long case or the operative stress of free tissue transfer.
  - Pedicled flaps should be considered when future microsurgery is planned and recipient vessels on the hand are limited.

B. First Web Space

- Goals of reconstruction: Allow the thumb to assume a position out of the plane of the fingers; allow the thumb to assume a position away from the fingers; allow the thumb to make contact with the fingers.

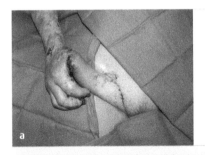 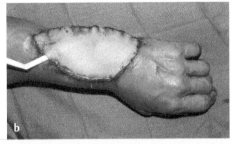

Fig. 19.10 Groin flap (pedicled and free).

1. Z-plasty

- Z-plasty utilizes interdigitating random pattern triangular flaps to lengthen and reorient scars.
- In designing the flaps, the total flap limb lengths should be roughly equal to the contracture length.
- Standard angles are used: A 60-degree angle results in 75% lengthening of the scar/contracture.
- To gain even greater length, each flap can be divided into two, to create "four-flap" Z-plasty:
  - A four-flap Z-plasty provides greater increase in length and depth than a two-flap Z-plasty.
- A "five-flap" Z-plasty can be created by incorporation of a V-Y advancement flap.

2. Skin Graft

- If there are no exposed vital structures (bone, tendon, nerve, or artery) a skin graft can be utilized to resurface the first web space.
- A full-thickness skin graft, more pliable and less prone to secondary contraction than a split-thickness graft, is preferred in this area.

3. PIA Flap

- This flap, as previously described, can usually reach the first web space:
  - This method of reconstruction avoids the need for microsurgery.
  - The donor defect is often resurfaced with skin graft and may be unsightly.
  - The flap may be hair bearing which might require depilation once healed.
  - Pedicle tension can be reduced by extending the wrist.

4. Free Lateral Arm Flap

- Usually harvested from the ipsilateral arm, this fasciocutaneous flap provides supple, often hairless skin to the first web space.
- The flap is supplied by the posterior radial collateral artery which is usually anastomosed to the radial artery at the "snuff box."
- Prior to harvest, the flap is oriented over the lateral aspect of the humerus, centered between the anterior and posterior compartments of the arm along a line from the deltoid to the lateral humeral epicondyle.
- The flap can be extended distal to the lateral epicondyle.
- The flap is harvested in a subfascial plane taking care to preserve the septum between the anterior and posterior compartments of the arm.
- The radial nerve (between the brachialis and brachioradialis) must be identified and protected.
- A bit bulkier than the PIA flap, the flap may require thinning at a second stage.

V. Forearm

- Goals of reconstruction: Soft tissue coverage of vital structures; minimization of scar; preservation of the aesthetic.
  - Consider a skin or fasciocutaneous flap if further surgeries are planned.

- Consider a skin or fasciocutaneous flap for distal forearm wounds where tendinous structures predominate and nerves are superficial.
  - Skin or fasciocutaneous flaps are robust and can withstand repeat elevation for revision surgeries.
- Skin graft should be considered for proximal, single-stage coverage requiring no further work.
  - Skin grafts are not robust and cannot withstand repeat elevation for revision surgeries.
- Pedicled or free flaps should be used if high quality tissue is desired:
  - The previously described pedicled flaps, including the PIA and radial forearm flaps, can be utilized to resurface vital structures in the forearm.
    - Either flap can be used in a "reverse" or "anterograde" fashion.
  - Free tissue transfer can allow for the coverage of large surface area and the selection of the tissue most appropriate for the wound
  - Muscle obliterates dead space and provides a nonbulky final contour:
    - Muscle can be difficult to re-elevate if future surgery is needed.
    - Large muscle (latissimus) can resurface a tremendous wound and has a pedicle long enough to position the anastomosis outside of the zone of injury.
    - Muscle can be transferred with motor nerve (latissimus or gracilis) to deliver function to an extremity with a motor deficit. This requires a working proximal motor nerve in good condition (e.g., AIN).
- Adjacent tissue rearrangement
  - There are a variety of local flaps which can be used for forearm wounds.
  - Local tissue has the benefit of excellent color and contour match.
  - The volar and dorsal skin laxity allows for harvest of random flaps (e.g., rhomboid flap and bilobed flap) with primary closure of the donor site.
  - Random pattern flaps should have a length:width ratio of 1:1 to ensure adequate perfusion via the subdermal plexus:
    - The survival of larger random pattern flaps can be improved by utilizing the "delay phenomenon" in which the skin cuts are initially made down to fascia but the flap is not elevated.
    - After 3 to 7 days, when the flap can be elevated, the "delay" will have opened "choke" vessels allowing for perfusion of the flap periphery.

VI. Elbow

- Goals of reconstruction: Supple elbow motion and coverage of vital structures:
  - The elbow must be supple enough to allow proper positioning of the hand in space.
  - The elbow should be supple enough to allow the hand to touch the face/mouth.
  - The skin overlying the olecranon should be durable and supple to prevent wear and pressure phenomena, without limiting motion.
- Pedicled radial forearm flap:
  - This flap, previously described as a "reverse" flap, can be raised as "anterograde" when the flap is based at the level of the distal volar forearm.
    - When elevated in this fashion, the arterial supply (proximal to distal) and venous drainage (distal to proximal) to the flap are considered physiologic.
  - The flap is raised in a distal to proximal fashion, freeing the radial artery from its interval between the FCR and BR.

- Mobilizing the radial artery proximally allows the flap to be transported to the elbow facilitating coverage of the olecranon or antecubital fossa as needed.
- Confirming adequate collateral flow to the hand should be confirmed prior to dividing the radial artery.
- PIA flap
  - This flap, previously described as a "reverse flap," can also be raised as "antero-grade" when the flap is based at the level of the distal dorsal forearm centered over the interval between the ECU and EDQ.
  - The flap is dissected subfascially, preserving the septum between the ECU and EDQ, in a distal to proximal fashion.
  - A leash of adipofascial tissue should be elevated with the flap to augment the blood supply and venous drainage.
  - Mobilizing the posterior interosseous artery proximally allows the flap to be transported to the elbow facilitating coverage of the olecranon or antecubital fossa as needed.
- Pedicled lateral arm flap
  - The lateral arm flap, previously described as a free flap, can be used in a pedicled fashion to allow for coverage of the olecranon or antecubital fossa.
    - The flap provides excellent color and skin quality match.
    - The flap, unless islandized, will require a debulking once it has incorporated into the surrounding soft tissues.
  - The flap is dissected in a proximal to distal fashion (protecting the radial nerve) and kept attached distally to preserve retrograde blood flow from the radial recurrent perforators.
  - The posterior cutaneous nerves of the arm and forearm have to be transected to mobilize the flap distally.
    - The sensory deficit over the lateral aspect of the elbow and forearm is usually well tolerated.
  - The donor site, if 6 cm wide or less, can usually be closed primarily.
  - Preoperative tissue expansion can allow for coverage of larger defects.

VII. Upper Arm

- Goals of reconstruction: Wound closure, avoidance of stiffness, and preservation of aesthetic:
  - Wounds at this level can often be closed either primarily, with a skin graft (split or full thickness) or with a local pedicled flap (e.g., rhomboid flap).
  - Regional flaps (e.g., pedicled latissimus dorsi flap) or free flaps should be considered for large wounds with exposed vital structures, those requiring obliteration of dead space or return of function, or those for which traditional methods of closure would result in stiffness or contracture.
- Pedicled latissimus dorsi flap:
  - Based off the thoracodorsal artery.
  - This flap provides a large muscle which can be used as a motorized flap to restore function (e.g., elbow flexion) or as a nonmotorized flap to resurface large deficits of tissue in the upper arm.
  - Though a skin paddle can be harvested with the flap, this is usually to act as a flap monitor.
    - A skin graft is often required to cover the flap.

- Little functional deficit from taking the latissimus muscle.
- This flap can reliably cover the shoulder and medial or lateral arm and can occasionally reach the antecubital fossa.
- If there is any tension on the pedicle, the flap should not be used in a pedicled fashion and instead, should be converted to a free flap.

References

[1] Elliot D, Moiemen NS. Composite graft replacement of digital tips. 1. Before 1850 and after 1950. J Hand Surg Br. 1997 June; 22(3):341–345.

[2] Moiemen NS, Elliot D. Composite graft replacement of digital tips. 2. A study in children. J Hand Surg Br. 1997 Jun;22(3):346–352.

[3] Eberlin KR, Busa K, Bae DS, Waters PM, Labow BI, Taghinia AH. Composite grafting for pediatric fingertip injuries. Hand (N Y) 2015;10(1):28–33

[4] Foucher G, Smith D, Pempinello C, Braun FM, Citron N. Homodigital neurovascular island flaps for digital pulp loss. J Hand Surg Br. 1989 May;14(2):204–208

[5] Gharb BB, Rampazzo A, Armijo BS, et al. Tranquilli-Leali or Atasoy flap: an anatomical cadaveric study. J Plast Reconstr Aesthet Surg 2010;63(4):681–685

[6] Jackson EA. The V-Y plasty in the treatment of fingertip amputations. Am Fam Physician. 2001 Aug 1;64 (3):455–458

[7] Smith KL, Elliot D. The extended Segmüller flap. Plast Reconstr Surg 2000;105(4):1334–1346

Suggested Readings

Moody L, Galvez MG, Chang J. Reconstruction of first web space contractures. J Hand Surg Am 2015;40(9):1892–1895, quiz 1896

Shepard GH. The use of lateral V-Y advancement flaps for fingertip reconstruction. J Hand Surg Am 1983;8(3):254–259

Taras JS, Sapienza A, Roach JB, Taras JP. Acellular dermal regeneration template for soft tissue reconstruction of the digits. J Hand Surg Am 2010;35(3):415–421

20 Vascular Pathology of the Hand and Upper Extremities, including Kienbock's Disease

Ariel Williams and Lauren Lee Smith

Abstract

Vascular pathology in the hand and upper extremity encompasses a broad range of conditions, some resulting in carpal osteonecrosis and mechanical wrist pain, others in insufficient blood flow to the digits with resultant ischemia and ulceration. Although hand surgeons have gained a far better understanding of the pathophysiology of these conditions over the last few decades, many mysteries remain.

This chapter provides an overview of the most notable vascular conditions affecting the hand, from the very common (Raynaud's disease) to the very rare (digital artery aneurysm). Specific subjects include Kienbock's disease, Preiser's disease, hypothenar hammer syndrome, Raynaud's phenomenon, thromboangiitis obliterans or "Buerger's disease," and digital artery aneurysm.

Keywords: Peripheral vascular disease, Kienbock's disease, Preiser's disease, avascular necrosis, hypothenar hammer, Raynaud's disease, thromboangiitis obliterans, aneurysm

I. Kienbock's Disease

A. Introduction

- Kienbock's disease = lunate osteonecrosis.
- Results in predictable sequence of lunate necrosis, fragmentation, and collapse, eventually leading to carpal malalignment and arthritis.
- Most commonly seen in 20- to 40-year-old males, although has been described in pediatric patients and older adults.
- Although it is less common, prognosis best in children and elderly.

B. Pathophysiology

- True cause unknown—likely multifactorial.
- A number of biomechanical and anatomic factors have been identified as playing a possible role although their true contribution is unknown:
  - History of repetitive wrist trauma.
  - Negative ulnar variance.
  - Decreased radial inclination.
  - Lunate geometry.
  - Differences in lunate vascularity.

C. Examination

- Dorsal wrist pain related to activity.
- Tenderness over lunate (palpate dorsally).
- Wrist swelling.

- Decreased wrist range of motion (ROM).
- Decreased grip strength.

D. Imaging

1. Radiographs

- Three views of wrist should be obtained.
- Radiographs demonstrate a predictable pattern of disease evolution over time.
- The Lichtman's classification is the most frequently used staging system (▶ Table 20.1). Stages 0 and IIIC have recently been added.
- Correct staging of the disease is critical to guide treatment choice.
- Stage II and stage III are distinguished by the collapse of the lunate in stage III.
- The scaphoid ring sign (▶ Fig. 20.1) and radioscaphoid angle (▶ Fig. 20.2) may be useful in differentiating between stages IIIA and IIIB.

2. Magnetic Resonance Imaging (MRI)

- May be performed with or without contrast.
- Changes correspond to Lichtman's staging system.
- Detects early disease while X-rays are still negative (Lichtman stage I):
  - Findings: Lunate signal decreases on T1 sequences, variable on T2 sequences.
- Gadolinium can be helpful. Unlike necrotic tissue, neovascular tissue enhances on T1 images when gadolinium is used. When observed, this may indicate a better prognosis for healing than when such enhancement does not occur.
- MRI can also demonstrate integrity of lunate cartilage shell.

3. Arthroscopy

- Can evaluate the articular surfaces of the lunate, radius, and capitate to support the decision to proceed with reconstructive versus salvage surgery.

Table 20.1 Lichtman's classification of Kienbock's disease

Stage	Radiographic findings
0	X-ray and MRI normal
I	X-ray normal; edema within lunate on MRI
II	Lunate sclerosis
IIIA	Lunate collapse without malalignment
IIIB	Lunate collapse; scaphoid malrotation and proximal capitate migration
IIIC	Lunate is fragmented or fractured in coronal plane
IV	Arthrosis

Abbreviation: MRI, magnetic resonance imaging.

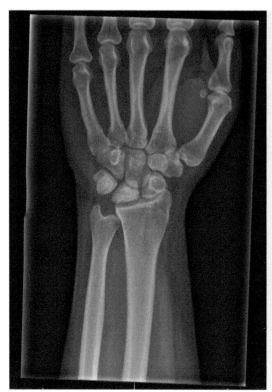

Fig. 20.1 Patient with stage IIIB Kienbock's disease and a scaphoid ring sign, which indicates flexion and malrotation of the scaphoid.

E. Treatment

- Treat children nonoperatively as outcomes are excellent.
- For adults, treatment depends on disease stage.
- Multiple treatment options exist. However, there is controversy regarding which procedures are best, especially in stage III disease.
- Nonsteroidal anti-inflammatory drug (NSAIDs), activity modification, and immobilization are all useful initial management at any stage.
- Surgical treatments include revascularization procedures, unloading procedures, and salvage procedures.
- Revascularization and unloading procedures are most effective in Lichtman stage 0, I, and II disease. They are less successful in stage III disease and contraindicated in stage IV disease.
- Revascularization procedures:
  - Aim to facilitate lunate recovery by restoring blood supply.
  - Distal radius core decompression:
    - Drill distal radius to increase local blood flow.
  - Lunate decompression:
    - Drill lunate to relieve venous congestion.
  - Vascularized bone grafts:
    - Pedicled: 4 and 5 extensor compartment artery or 2nd or 3rd dorsal metacarpal arteries.
    - Free: Vascularized iliac crest, medial femoral trochlea.

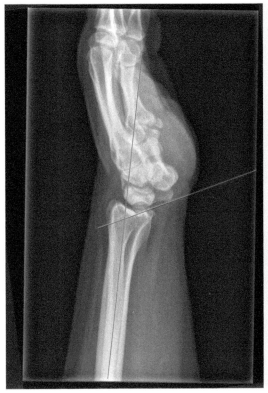

Fig. 20.2 Measurement of the radioscaphoid angle (RS) in a patient with Kienbock's disease. A radioscaphoid angle of greater than 60 degrees is an indicator of stage IIIB disease.

- ○ An unloading procedure can be performed at the same time to optimize conditions for lunate recovery. Alternatively, K-wires or an external fixator can be used to temporarily unload the lunate while healing takes place.
- Unloading procedures:
  - ○ Aim to facilitate lunate recovery by altering biomechanical forces.
  - ○ Radial shortening osteotomy:
    - – Ulnar negative patients only.
  - ○ Capitate shortening osteotomy:
    - – Patients who are ulnar neutral or ulnar positive.
- Salvage procedures:
  - ○ Lichtman stages III and IV.
  - ○ Aim to reduce pain once the lunate is no longer viable.
    - – Procedure choice based upon patient's age and extent of surrounding deformity, arthrosis.
  - ○ Proximal row carpectomy.
  - ○ Partial wrist arthrodesis (lunate excision scaphocapitate fusion or scaphotrapezio-trapezoid [STT] fusion).
  - ○ Pyrocarbon lunate replacement.
  - ○ Wrist fusion or arthroplasty.
    - – Pan-carpal arthrosis.

II. Preiser's Disease

A. Introduction

- Idiopathic avascular necrosis of the scaphoid:
  - Distinct from post-traumatic osteonecrosis observed in the context of scaphoid nonunion.
  - However, patients may have some history of trauma.
- Although idiopathic avascular necrosis has been reported in all the carpal bones, the scaphoid is the second most commonly affected (the lunate is first).
- Despite this, Preiser's disease is rare.
- Average age of onset is in the fourth decade of life.
- More commonly affects dominant side.

B. Pathophysiology

- Scaphoid's limited blood supply (retrograde flow) is a predisposing factor.
- Repetitive microtrauma, steroid use, chemotherapy, collagen vascular disease, and other factors may contribute in some cases.
- Two patterns are seen:
  - Type I: Entire scaphoid involved.
  - Type II: Only proximal pole involved.
- Type I has worse prognosis.

C. Examination

- Dorsoradial wrist pain.
- Wrist swelling.
- Loss of wrist ROM.
- Diminished grip strength.

D. Imaging

1. Radiographs

- Three views of wrist.
- Scaphoid sclerosis and fragmentation as disease progresses but with no evidence of fracture.

2. MRI

- Signal changes similar to the lunate in Kienbock's disease (▶ Fig. 20.3).
- Evaluation for complete versus partial involvement (type I vs. type II).

3. Computed Tomography (CT)

- May be useful to rule out fracture.

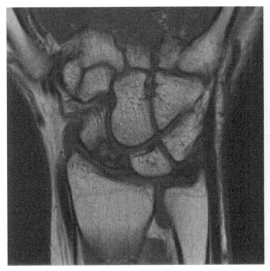

Fig. 20.3 A patient with type II Preiser's disease, with decreased signal on T1-weighted MRI of the proximal scaphoid pole only.

E. Treatment

1. Nonoperative

- Immobilization, activity modification, nonsteroidal anti-inflammatory medications, and steroid injection.
- Results are varied; progression in early stages is common.

2. Operative

- Revascularization procedures:
  - Prior to scaphoid fragmentation/fracture.
  - Pedicled vascularized graft from 1, 2 intercompartmental supraretinacular artery or pronator quadratus.
  - Free vascularized graft from medial femoral condyle:
    - Can also be utilized for scaphoid reconstruction once proximal pole collapse has occurred.
- Salvage procedures:
  - Arthroscopic debridement.
  - Scaphoid excision and silicone replacement.
  - Proximal row carpectomy.
  - Scaphoid excision with four-corner fusion.
  - Wrist arthrodesis or arthroplasty when pancarpal arthrosis is present.

III. Hypothenar Hammer Syndrome

A. Introduction

- The ulnar artery is the most common site of upper extremity aneurysm.
- In hypothenar hammer syndrome, the ulnar artery becomes thrombosed at Guyon's canal due to closed trauma to the palm of the hand.

- Most often this is due to repeated trauma (e.g., manual laborers who repeatedly use the palm as a hammer), although also can be seen after a single event.
- More common in males with a ratio of 9:1.
- Dominant limb most often affected.

B. Pathophysiology

- Ulnar artery and nerve lie superficial in the hypothenar area, directly radial to hook of hamate.
- Repetitive trauma compresses the ulnar artery against hook of the hamate, eventually resulting in arterial thrombosis, aneurysm, and/or embolization.
- This may eventually result in vascular insufficiency.

C. Examination

- Pain in the hypothenar eminence.
- Cold sensitivity, paresthesia in ring and small fingers.
- Weakness in ulnar nerve distribution.
- Pulsatile mass, if aneurysm present.
- Splinter hemorrhages.
- Pallor, gangrene, mottling, and blanching over ulnar two digits.
- Allen's test positive.

D. Imaging

- Doppler ultrasound
  - May show thrombosis and aneurysmal dilation of the ulnar artery at the hypothenar eminence.
- Digital brachial index: Will be decreased in the ulnar-most digits
- Angiogram
  - Torturous appearing "corkscrew" ulnar artery.
  - Aneurysm or arterial occlusion at the hook of the hamate.

E. Treatment

1. Nonoperative

- Only if there is no threat to digital viability.
- Avoidance of aggravating activity.
- Smoking cessation.
- Calcium channel blockers.
- Anticoagulation and antiplatelet agents.
- Symptomatic management.

2. Operative

- If nonsurgical management fails or if there is threat of tissue loss.
- Catheter-directed thrombolysis.
- Excision of involved segment and repair/reconstruction.

- If end-to-end repair not possible, reconstruction can be performed with either vein or arterial interposition graft or with bypass.
- Leriche's sympathectomy:
  - Ligation and excision of diseased segment.
  - Inflow from radial artery must be sufficient to maintain good circulation in absence of ulnar artery.
  - Results in local sympathectomy.

IV. Raynaud's Phenomenon

A. Introduction

- Transient, recurrent pain and color changes in the digits in response to exposure to cold temperature:
  - Acral color change from white (ischemic) to blue (cyanotic) to red (reperfused).
  - Can also be triggered by stress.
  - Although digits most commonly involved, can also affect toes, ears, and/or nipples.
- More common in women.
- Onset usually in early adulthood.
- Raynaud's disease versus Raynaud's syndrome:
  - Raynaud's disease (primary Raynaud's syndrome) has no underlying cause. The course is benign. Irreversible tissue changes do not occur. It is generally symmetric.
  - Raynaud's syndrome (secondary Raynaud's syndrome) occurs in patients with collagen vascular disease. It is most commonly associated with scleroderma. Patients may develop digital trophic changes, chronic ulcers and gangrene. It can be asymmetric.

B. Pathophysiology

- Digital ischemia due to exaggerated cold-induced vasospasm.
- A number of molecular regulators of vascular tone have been identified that may mediate this process, such as nitric oxide and the renin-angiotensin system.

C. Examination

- Patients should be questioned regarding risk factors and symptoms that would raise concern for collagen vascular disease.
- If there is concern for collagen vascular disease, laboratory workup or rheumatology referral should be undertaken to evaluate this further.
- Peripheral pulses.
- Allen's test.
- Skin should be inspected for any trophic changes.
- Cold simulation testing: A temperature probe is taped to the patient's fingers. The hand is immersed in ice water and then removed. After removing the hand from the water, the temperature normally returns to baseline within 15 minutes. If it takes longer than 20 minutes to return to baseline, the results are consistent with Raynaud's.

D. Imaging

- Although not indicated in most cases of primary Raynaud's phenomenon, in patients with chronic ulcerations, angiogram should be considered to look for occlusive small or large vessel disease.

E. Treatment

- Supportive measures suffice in most cases:
  - Education is key.
  - Gloves.
  - Keeping core body warm to reduce peripheral vasoconstriction.
  - Avoidance of cold temperatures, rewarming techniques such as motion and warm water.
  - Smoking cessation, avoidance of medications that may promote vasoconstriction.
  - For patients with secondary Raynaud's phenomenon, the underlying collagen vascular disease must be addressed.
- Medical management:
  - Calcium channel blockers are first line (nifedipine, amlodipine).
  - Phosphodiesterase-5 inhibitors such as sildenafil.
  - Topical nitrates.
- Injections of botulinum toxin.
- Surgical sympathectomy:
  - Reserved for those with chronic ulcerations refractory to other measures.

V. Thromboangiitis Obliterans (Buerger's Disease)

A. Introduction

- Segmental inflammatory vasculitis of small- and medium-sized arteries, veins, and nerves of the upper and lower extremities of predominantly male tobacco users.
- Results in nonatherosclerotic vascular occlusion.
- Prevalence declining, linked to rates of tobacco usage.

B. Epidemiology

- Male:female ratio is 3:1.
- Typically affects patients < 45 years old.
- Affects current or past tobacco users exclusively (most commonly heavy smokers although also those who chew tobacco).

C. Pathophysiology

- Etiology unknown.
- Possible association with periodontal bacteria has been raised.
- Unlike atherosclerosis and other forms of vasculitis, architecture of the vessel wall is usually intact.
- Three histopathologic phases:
  - Acute: Inflammatory thrombi appear.

○ Subacute: Thrombi organize.
○ Chronic: Vessel fibrosis occurs.

D. History

- Initial claudication of distal extremities progresses to ischemic rest pain.
- Ulcerations of toes and fingers develop.
- Often, all four limbs are affected.
- Superficial thrombophlebitis frequent.

E. Examination

- Acral ulcerations.
- Gangrene.
- Diminished/absent pulses.
- Positive Allen's test.

F. Imaging

- Four limb segmental arterial Doppler pressures.
- Toe and finger plethysmography.
- Digital plethysmography.
- Arteriography useful in treatment planning and when diagnosis is in doubt.
  ○ Will show small and medium size vessel occlusion with abundant collateral circulation:
    – Collaterals take on tortuous appearance: "Corkscrew" vessels.

G. Treatment

- Tobacco cessation is mainstay of care and for many patients will avoid amputation:
  ○ Patient education.
  ○ Pharmacotherapy:
    – Nicotine substitutes should be avoided as they may prevent disease remission.
  ○ Smoking cessation groups.
- Medical management
  ○ Although vasodilators are sometimes used, their efficacy is not clear.
- Operative
  ○ Amputation of nonviable digits is the most common intervention.
  ○ In most cases, revascularization not an option due to lack of a patent distal vessel, although it can be attempted in rare cases where a target is identified.
  ○ Postoperative patency rates are higher in patients who stop smoking preoperatively.
  ○ Role of Botox and surgical sympathectomy is controversial.

VI. Digital Artery Aneurysm

A. Introduction

- Aneurysms of the digital artery are quite rare.

- Ulnar artery aneurysms are more common.
- Any digit can be affected.
- Not typically associated with complications of rupture or hemorrhage.

B. Pathophysiology

- May be true aneurysms or false aneurysms.
  - True aneurysms:
    - Weakened vessel wall becomes focally dilated.
    - Generally arise from blunt trauma.
  - False aneurysms:
    - Rupture of arterial wall resulting in leakage of blood and formation of contained thrombus outside vessel wall.
    - Generally arise from penetrating trauma.

C. Examination

- Firm mass in line with digital neurovascular bundle.
- May or may not be pulsatile.
- Often tender.
- Digital Allen's test can be helpful in assessing patency of involved digital artery and adequacy of collateral circulation.

D. Imaging

- MRI will show mass arising from or adjacent to digital neurovascular bundle.
- Duplex ultrasound will show vascular flow, differentiating from solid tumor or cyst.
- Angiography is the gold standard, although supplanted to some extent by the above techniques.

E. Treatment

- Excision with ligation versus arterial reconstruction:
  - In most cases, the collateral circulation will provide adequate flow without need for reconstruction, although cold intolerance can be an issue with single vessel perfusion.
  - If reconstruction is undertaken, this can be accomplished with interposition vein graft.

Suggested Readings

Abouzahr MK, Coppa LM, Boxt LM. Aneurysms of the digital arteries: a case report and literature review. J Hand Surg Am. 1997; 22(2):311–314

Afshar A, Tabrizi A. Avascular necrosis of the carpal bones other than Kienböck disease. J Hand Surg Am. 2020; 45(2):148–152

Allan CH, Joshi A, Lichtman DM. Kienbock's disease: diagnosis and treatment. J Am Acad Orthop Surg. 2001; 9(2):128–136

Dargon PT, Landry GJ. Buerger's disease. Ann Vasc Surg. 2012; 26(6):871–880

Goldfarb CA, Hsu J, Gelberman RH, Boyer MI. The Lichtman classification for Kienböck's disease: an assessment of reliability. J Hand Surg Am. 2003; 28(1):74–80

Ho PK, Weiland AJ, McClinton MA, Wilgis EFS. Aneurysms of the upper extremity. J Hand Surg Am. 1987; 12(1):39–46

Hui-Chou HG, McClinton MA. Current options for treatment of hypothenar hammer syndrome. Hand Clin. 2015; 31 (1):53–62

Lenoir H, Coulet B, Lazerges C, Mares O, Croutzet P, Chammas M. Idiopathic avascular necrosis of the scaphoid: 10 new cases and a review of the literature. Indications for Preiser's disease. Orthop Traumatol Surg Res. 2012; 98 (4):390–397

Lichtman DM, Pientka WF, II, Bain GI. Kienböck disease: a new algorithm for the 21st century. J Wrist Surg. 2017; 6 (1):2–10

Lin JD, Strauch RJ. Preiser disease. J Hand Surg Am. 2013; 38(9):1833–1834

Marques E. Ulnar artery thrombosis: hypothenar hammer syndrome. J Am Coll Surg. 2008; 206(1):188–189

Neumeister MW. Botulinum toxin type A in the treatment of Raynaud's phenomenon. J Hand Surg Am. 2010; 35 (12):2085–2092

Olin JW. Thromboangiitis obliterans (Buerger's disease). N Engl J Med. 2000; 343(12):864–869

Sokolow C, Theron P,, Saffar P. Preiser's disease. J Am Soc Surg Hand. 2004; 4(2):103–108

Stringer T, Femia AN. Raynaud's phenomenon: current concepts. Clin Dermatol. 2018; 36(4):498–507

Wolfe SW, Hotchkiss RN, Pederson WC, Kozin SH, Cohen MS, Green DP. Green's Operative hand surgery. 7th ed. Philadelphia, PA: Elsevier; 2017

21 Digital Replantation and Revascularization

Alexandra Tilt and Mitchell A. Pet

Abstract

Digital replantation and revascularization are technically challenging procedures which present with little warning. In this time-pressured situation, attention to Advanced Trauma Life Support (ATLS) protocol and a meticulous medical history are critical for determining operative candidacy. Traditional indications for replantation are reviewed in this chapter, with additional discussion of how indications have evolved in modern practice. Important elements of the preoperative discussion and informed consent are outlined. Once the decision to pursue replantation has been made, a directed and efficient operative plan is critical for success. This chapter provides a detailed summary of the authors' preferred technique for single finger digital replantation, and commentary on special considerations for thumb and multiple digit replantation.

Keywords: Digital replantation, microsurgery, indications for replantation

I. Patient Evaluation

- Advanced Trauma Life Support (ATLS)
  - First priority is identification of other injuries; amputation is a distractor.
- History
  - Time and mechanism of injury.
  - Occupation, handedness, and social situation.
  - Complete medical history to elucidate comorbidities in anticipation of general anesthesia and hospitalization.
- Physical examination
  - Incomplete and complete amputations:
    - Level of injury and degree of contamination.
    - Radiographs of hand and amputated part.
  - Incomplete amputations:
    - Color and capillary refill, doppler assessment of each digital vessel.
    - Test sensation in each digital nerve distribution prior to any local anesthesia.
    - Active tendon examination and/or passive tenodesis.
- Preoperative testing
  - Complete blood count (CBC), basic metabolic panel (BMP), prothrombin time (PT)/international normalized ratio (INR), consider type and screen.
  - Electrocardiogram (EKG) and chest X-ray based upon medical history.

II. The Amputated Part

- In the field and during transport, an amputated part should be wrapped with saline-moistened gauze, placed in a plastic bag, and then put on ice.
  - Do not submerge the part or put it directly on ice.
- Digits can tolerate up to 12 hours of warm or 24 hours of cold ischemia for successful replantation or revascularization.[1]

- Bleeding vessels should be controlled with direct pressure or a gentle compressive dressing. Tourniquet, cautery, and ligation are discouraged in the absence of persistent and dangerous hemorrhage.
- Discard nothing. Unreplantable digits may still be used for spare parts (nerve, skin, bone, or tendon graft).

III. Indications and Decision-Making

A. Traditional Indications for Replantation

- Thumb amputation.
- Multiple digit amputation.
- Partial or total hand through the palm, wrist, forearm, elbow, or above.
- Almost any part in a child:
  - Technically more difficult, but excellent functional results when successful.
- Single digit amputation distal to the flexor digitorum superficialis (FDS) insertion:
  - Zone I outcomes are superior to Zone II.[2]

B. Traditional Contraindications to Replantation

- Severely crushed or mangled parts.
- Amputations at multiple levels.
- Amputations in patients with other serious injuries/diseases.
- Severe atherosclerotic disease.
- Prolonged warm ischemia.
- Mentally or medically unstable patient.
- Individual finger amputation in an adult at a level proximal to the FDS insertion.

C. Indications in Modern Practice

- The decision to perform replantation/revascularization in cases of single non-thumb digital amputation is shared by the patient and surgeon. This decision process is complex, and is influenced by numerous factors that must be weighed in each individual circumstance.
  - Mechanism, level, and ischemia time.
  - Age and medical comorbidities
    - Risk of prolonged anesthesia and hospitalization should be a primary concern.
  - Physical and occupational demands
    - Manual laborers will likely return to work sooner with revision amputation compared with replantation and should be counseled as such.
  - Social factors.
  - Cultural and personal values.
  - Availability of postreplantation care and occupational therapy.

IV. Informed Consent

- Informed consent should include replantation with possible nerve allograft or autograft, vein autograft, skin autograft, and revision amputation.
- The alternative of revision amputation should be specifically discussed.

- Important disclosures:
  - Replantation is effort-intensive, and may necessitate prolonged time out of work.
  - Anesthetic and hospital-associated complications are possible.
  - Attempted replantation is not always successful. Postoperative digital necrosis requiring amputation is possible.
  - Leech therapy may be indicated, and it may necessitate blood transfusion.
  - Postoperative stiffness and subnormal sensation are likely.
  - Secondary surgery may be recommended.

V. Surgical Technique

A. Preparation

- Both the part and hand should be prepped using iodine, and then copiously irrigated.
- With the tourniquet down, gentle pressure is applied to the dorsum of the hand/ finger, just proximal to the amputation. Sites of venous bleeding are marked on the skin, and the marking is transferred to the adjacent site on the amputated part. This facilitates vein identification later in the case.
- In most cases, it is our preference to forego back-table dissection in favor of immediate osteosynthesis.
  - In our opinion, restoring the native gross anatomy of the hand makes all subsequent dissection more intuitive and efficient. Additionally, delaying neurovascular dissection until after osteosynthesis reduces the risk that skeletonized neurovascular structures become wrapped around K-wires.

B. Skeletal Shortening and Osteosynthesis

- Skeletal shortening and osteosynthesis should be performed before raising the tourniquet if possible.
- Bone is shortened to facilitate primary nerve and vessel coaptation outside the zone of injury. If possible, preferentially shorten the amputated part to preserve proximal skeletal length in case of replant failure.
- Fixation should be simple and fast. Extensive soft tissue stripping is avoided. Careful attention is given to avoid trauma to the neurovascular bundles and dorsal veins. K-wires placed in an antegrade/retrograde fashion and/or interosseous wires are recommended (▶ Fig. 21.1). External fixation using a 1-cc syringe and 0.045 K-wires is useful if the fracture is extensively comminuted. Transarticular trauma should be treated with shortening and arthrodesis.

C. Exposure

- Exsanguinate the limb and raise the tourniquet.
- Skin incision is based upon surgeon preference, but should take into account the orientation of the traumatic laceration. We generally prefer short mid-lateral incisions on the finger, with transition to a Bruner pattern proximal to the metacarpophalangeal joint crease. Avoid the web space.
- The tendon sheath should be exposed at this point, but the neurovascular bundles should not yet be dissected.

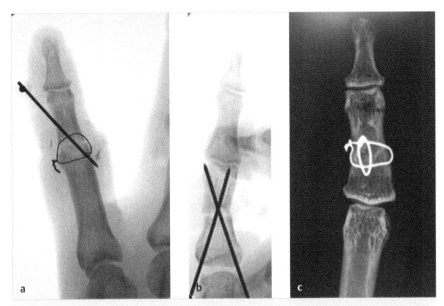

Fig. 21.1 Three examples of appropriate osteosynthesis in replantation. (a) After transarticular amputation of the index finger a primary fusion was accomplished using a single coronal plane interosseous wire and an oblique K-wire. (b) After amputation of the small finger through the proximal phalanx diaphysis, osteosynthesis was accomplished with crossed K-wires. These were first placed into the amputated part in an anterograde direction before being driven retrograde into the proximal fragment. (c) After middle finger amputation through the middle phalanx, osteosynthesis was accomplished using 90–90 interosseous wires.

D. Tendon Repair

- Flexor tenorrhaphy
  - Tendon(s) can usually be grasped within the tendon sheath using a Carroll tendon retriever or Jacobsen clamp. If this is not possible, a counter-incision at the A1 pulley or carpal tunnel may be necessary. Once retrieved, the tendon should be transfixed with a 25 gauge needle through the skin, securing it out to length.
  - Epitendinous and locking core repair of the flexor digitorum profundus or flexor pollicus longus is recommended.
  - In zone II consider repairing only one slip of FDS, or omitting FDS repair altogether.
- Extensor tenorrhaphy
  - Lift dorsal skin off the vein/adipose tissue with a scalpel.
  - Separate this tissue from underlying extensor tendon.
  - Repair using figure-of-eight sutures.

E. Neurovascular Bundle

- Carefully isolate radial and ulnar neurovascular bundles both proximally and distally, then separate artery and nerve. Tag each structure with a micro-clip at its very end.
- Arterial preparation and anastomosis.

○ Evaluate proximal and distal arterial stumps and flush with heparinized saline. Each end should be serially trimmed until the vessel is without evidence of injury. Look for intimal delamination and "cobwebbing" within the lumen. These are perhaps the most subtle signs of unresected injury.

○ One digital artery is sufficient for revascularization; repairing both may lead to venous congestion. In general, the ulnar digital artery of the thumb and index finger and the radial digital artery of the small and ring fingers will be larger.

○ Secure the vessel ends in a small, atraumatic double clamp and repair using 9–0 or 10–0 nylon microsuture. If tensionless primary coaptation is not possible, take vein graft from volar wrist (▶ Fig. 21.2), and interpose this in a reverse orientation.

○ Nerve coaptation
– Each nerve end is serially excised until healthy fascicles are visualized.
– Coaptation is done with 9–0 nylon microsuture. If tensionless primary coaptation is not possible, use allograft or posterior interosseous nerve autograft.

• Venous anastomosis
○ Make note of dorsal veins marked during preparation. This should aid in prompt identification. Tack back dorsal skin that has previously been raised off the dorsal adipose tissue.

○ Isolate proximal and distal dorsal veins and secure the vessel ends in a small atraumatic double clamp. Anastomose using 10–0 or 11–0 nylon microsuture. Back-wall technique is often necessary.

○ Repairing at least two veins has been linked to improved outcomes.[3]

F. Closure and Dressing

• Minimal primary closure should be performed. A few loose absorbable sutures may be used.

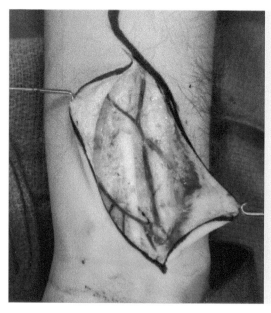

Fig. 21.2 In cases where bridging graft is necessary for digital arterial reconstruction, appropriate size veins can be easily harvested from the distal volar forearm.

- Copious antibiotic ointment should be placed over open incisions. It is acceptable to place this directly on top of neurovascular structures. Full-thickness skin graft is another option.
- A very loose and highly padded split should be applied. It should be open distally to facilitate postoperative monitoring.

VI. Special Situations

A. Thumb Replantation

- The pronated and radially abducted posture of the thumb makes repair of its ulnar digital artery difficult. This problem can be mitigated by extending the proximal arterial stump with a vein graft via a dorsal approach prior to reapproximating the amputated part. The amputated thumb is prepared with two longitudinal intramedullary K-wires, but when it is brought onto the field it is provisionally fixated using only one of these (▶ Fig. 21.3a). The thumb is then hypersupinated to facilitate the anastomosis. Only after a patent arterial anastomosis has been confirmed is the thumb pronated into an anatomic position and the second K-wire advanced proximally (▶ Fig. 21.3b).
- In cases where the proximal arterial stump is not suitable for anastomosis, vein grafting to the snuff box may be indicated. However, it should be kept in mind that the snuff box may need to be re-accessed for toe transfer if the replantation is not successful.

B. Multiple Digital Replantation

- When all injured digits have similar importance and probability of success, simultaneous replantation should be done structure-by-structure (not digit-by-digit).
- When multiple injured digits have varied relative importance and probability of success, replantation should proceed sequentially by part in order of importance.

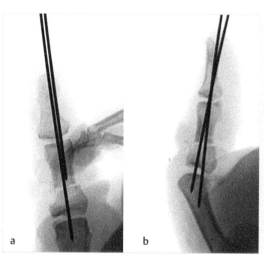

Fig. 21.3 The amputated thumb is prepared with two longitudinal intramedullary K-wires, but when it is brought onto the field it is provisionally fixated using only one of these (a). The thumb is then hypersupinated to facilitate the anastomosis. Only after a patent arterial anastomosis has been accomplished is the thumb then pronated into an anatomic position and the second K-wire advanced proximally (b).

C. Dysvascular but Nonamputated Parts

- Increased likelihood of survival and potentially superior outcomes have been shown when compared to complete amputations.[4] Indications for revascularization should be liberal.
- Even small skin bridges offer an enormous advantage by providing substantial venous drainage in the subdermal plexus.

VII. Postoperative Management

- Forced air warming blanket around splint.
- Limb elevation.
- Aspirin 325 mg orally per day.
- Subcutaneous heparin for deep vein thrombosis (DVT) prophylaxis.
- Caffeine-free diet, no nicotine, and volume expansion to avoid vasospasm.
- Monitoring should be based upon what salvage interventions would be offered for vascular compromise. If reoperation for arterial compromise would be considered, then hourly doppler and color checks are appropriate. If leech therapy would be offered for venous congestion, then hourly color checks are appropriate. We do not generally offer re-operation for salvage of a failing non-thumb single digit replant.
- After thumb or multiple digit replantation, we prefer inpatient management for at least 5 days. For single non-thumb digits, discharge is generally between 3 and 5 days after surgery, based upon patient's comfort and surgeon's preference.

VIII. Rehabilitation

- Early active short-arc motion should begin as soon as the wounds are healed, usually between 2 and 3 weeks postoperatively. Without aggressive rehabilitation, intractable stiffness is nearly uniform. Flexor tenolysis is often necessary to achieve satisfactory active motion.

References

[1] Lin C-H, Aydyn N, Lin Y-T, Hsu C-T, Lin C-H, Yeh J-T. Hand and finger replantation after protracted ischemia (more than 24 hours). Ann Plast Surg. 2010; 64(3):286–290

[2] Urbaniak JR, Roth JH, Nunley JA, Goldner RD, Koman LA. The results of replantation after amputation of a single finger. J Bone Joint Surg Am. 1985; 67(4):611–619

[3] Waikakul S, Sakkarnkosol S, Vanadurongwan V, Un-nanuntana A. Results of 1018 digital replantations in 552 patients. Injury. 2000; 31(1):33–40

[4] Soucacos PN, Beris AE, Touliatos AS, Korobilias AB, Gelalis J, Sakas G. Complete versus incomplete nonviable amputations of the thumb: comparison of the survival rate and functional results. Acta Orthop Scand Suppl. 1995; 264:16–18

22 Compartment Syndrome

Eric Lukosius and Kenneth F. Taylor

Abstract
Compartment syndrome in the upper extremity is a rare but potentially devastating condition resulting from a wide variety of insults that cause expansion of muscle fascial compartments. If inadequately treated in a timely fashion, resulting tissue ischemia may result in muscle and other soft tissue necrosis. Diagnosis is largely based on clinical suspicion but several ancillary studies serve to confirm its presence. Treatment involves surgically decompressing involved muscle tissue through appropriate fascial incisions.

Keywords: Compartment syndrome, fasciotomy, forearm, hand, trauma

I. Definition

- Compartment syndrome: Elevation of interstitial pressure in a closed fascial compartment, causing the perfusion gradient to fall below a critical value, leading to ischemia of the tissues within this confined space.[1]

II. Pathophysiology

- Increased compartment pressures lead to increased venous outflow obstruction. Resulting increased capillary permeability through changes in oncotic pressure promotes further increase in compartment expansion. Once high enough, arterial obstruction occurs and leads to decreased tissue oxygenation. This ischemic state is initially reversible.[2]

III. Etiology

- Trauma: Examples include distal radius fracture, crush injury, gunshot, and animal bite.
  - Most frequent cause of acute compartment syndrome.
  - High proportion of postfracture compartment syndrome occurs after fixation.[3]
- External compression
  - Examples: Tight casts, dressings, and wraps.
- Fluid extravasation
  - Examples: Intravenous (IV) fluids, anticoagulation, bleeding disorders, and vascular injury.
- Burns: Compression from circumferential eschar and increased tissue edema.[4]
- Exertional (chronic) compartment syndrome:
  - Exercise-induced, reversible increases in pressure within fascial compartments which usually resolves without permanent sequelae when the activity ceases.
  - Most typical in rigorous repetitive activity (rowers, swimmers, manual laborers).
  - In presence of anomalous muscle; examples include extensor digitorum brevis manus and reversed palmaris longus.

○ Additional diagnostic studies—dynamic compartment pressure measurements, magnetic resonance imaging, and near infrared spectroscopy.[5]

IV. Symptoms

- Pain out of proportion to physical examination.
- Increasing pain medication requirement.

V. Physical Examination

- Pain with passive stretch: Most sensitive.[1]
- Paresthesia and hypoesthesia.
- Paralysis.
- Palpable swelling.
- Peripheral pulses absent.

VI. Compartment Measures

- Especially useful in obtunded or otherwise unreliable patients.
- Side-port needles and slit catheters—more accurate than straight needles.[6]
- Diagnostic criteria:
  ○ Absolute value: Absolute value >30 mm Hg indicative of compartment syndrome.
  ○ Differential value: Measurement within 30 mm Hg of diastolic blood pressure.

VII. Treatment Options

- Serial examination: Appropriate if symptoms are early and patient can be closely monitored.
- Compartment release: If worsening on clinical examination, not expected to improve, prophylactic in the setting of reperfusion injury after revascularization/replantation, or patient expecting long transportation.[7]
- Three forearm compartments: Some consider pronator quadratus (PQ) to have its own compartment:
  ○ Volar (flexor digitorum profundus [FCR], flexor digitorum superficialis [FDS], flexor digitorum profundus [FDP], pronator teres [PT], flexor carpi ulnaris [FCU], PQ).
  ○ Dorsal (extensor digitorum communis [EDC], extensor indicis propius [EIP], extensor digiti quinti [EDQ], extensor carpi ulnaris [ECU], Supinator).
  ○ Mobile wad (brachialis [BR], extensor carpi radialis brevis [ECRB], extensor carpi radialis longus [ECRL]).
- Hand compartments:[8]
  ○ Carpal tunnel.
  ○ Thenar.
  ○ Hypothenar.
  ○ Intrinsic: Dorsal, palmar, and adductor.
- Emergent fasciotomies of all involved compartments:
  ○ Debride all devitalized structures to prevent postoperative infection.
  ○ Volar forearm incision.[9]

- Curvilinear incision starts just radial to FCU at wrist and extends proximally to medial epicondyle (▶ Fig. 22.1).
- Decompress the lacertus fibrosus, PQ, superficial and deep flexors.
- Can extend incision distally to include the carpal tunnel.
- Release of the volar compartments often results in decompression of the dorsal compartments through the same incision.[1]
  - Dorsal forearm incision
    - Longitudinal to mid-distal third of the forearm.
    - Identify and preserve the extensor retinaculum.
  - Hand incisions
    - Dorsal hand incisions: Over index and ring metacarpals to release intrinsic compartments (▶ Fig. 22.2).
    - Palmar hand incisions: Thenar, hypothenar, and carpal tunnel (extended) (▶ Fig. 22.3).
- Postoperative care
  - Skin incisions: Typically left open.
  - Dressing: Wet to dry dressing with or without tension device; wound vacuum-assisted closure (VAC).
  - Elevate extremity: Consider functional orthosis and early range of motion (ROM).
  - Multiple debridements: May be required before closure.
  - Delayed closure:
    - May require skin grafting for complete closure.
    - Avoid excessive tension or additional trauma to skin to prevent further ischemic damage.

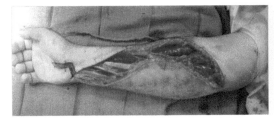

Fig. 22.1 Incision for release of volar forearm compartment.

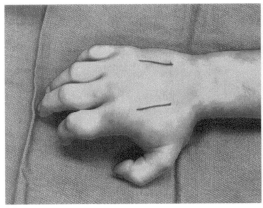

Fig. 22.2 Proposed incision for dorsal hand compartment release.

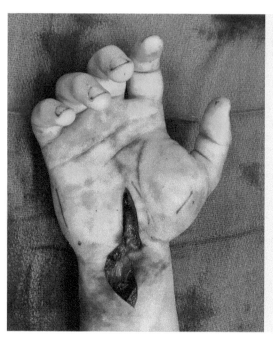

Fig. 22.3 Palmar hand compartment release incisions with extended carpal tunnel.

VIII. Adverse Outcomes

- Most common in unrecognized cases or insufficient treatment.
- Volkmann's ischemic contracture: Deep volar musculature at greatest risk.
- Neurologic deficit: Distal to point of compression.
- Infection: Secondary to necrotic tissue.
- Amputation: May be necessary to perform complete debridement or as a result of functional loss.

References

[1] Prasarn ML, Ouellette EA. Acute compartment syndrome of the upper extremity. J Am Acad Orthop Surg. 2011; 19(1):49–58

[2] Tollens T, Janzing H, Broos P. The pathophysiology of the acute compartment syndrome. Acta Chir Belg. 1998; 98(4):171–175

[3] Bodansky D, Doorgakant A, Alsousou J, et al. Acute compartment syndrome: do guidelines for diagnosis and management make a difference? Injury. 2018; 49(9):1699–1702

[4] Malic CC, Hernon C, Austin O, Phipps A. Scalded and swollen-beware the underlying compartment syndrome. Burns. 2006; 32(4):504–506

[5] Liu B, Barrazueta G, Ruchelsman DE. Chronic exertional compartment syndrome in athletes. J Hand Surg Am. 2017; 42(11):917–923

[6] Boody AR, Wongworawat MD. Accuracy in the measurement of compartment pressures: a comparison of three commonly used devices. J Bone Joint Surg Am. 2005; 87(11):2415–2422

[7] Kragh JF, Jr, Dubick MA, Aden JK, III, et al. U.S. military experience from 2001 to 2010 with extremity fasciotomy in war surgery. Mil Med. 2016; 181(5):463–468

[8] DiFelice A, Jr, Seiler JG, 3rd, Whitesides TE, Jr. The compartments of the hand: an anatomic study. J Hand Surg Am. 1998; 23(4):682–686

[9] Kistler JM, Ilyas AM, Thoder JJ. Forearm compartment syndrome: evaluation and management. Hand Clin. 2018; 34(1):53–60

23 Tumors of the Hand

Samir Sabharwal and Sophia Anne Strike

Abstract

Hand tumors comprise benign and malignant soft tissue and bony lesions. Thorough evaluation—generally comprising history and physical examination, plain radiography and cross-sectional imaging, and biopsy—is necessary to guide appropriate treatment. Of the benign pathologies, ganglion cysts, epidermal inclusion cysts, and tenosynovial giant cell tumors are the most common soft tissue lesions, and enchondromas are the most common bony lesions. Of the malignancies, epithelioid and synovial sarcomas are the most common soft tissue lesions and chondrosarcomas are the most common bony lesions. Benign lesions may be treated with observation or marginal/intralesional excision. Malignancies mandate wide resection and multidisciplinary oncologic care.

Keywords: Biopsy, local recurrence, wide resection, observation, ganglion cyst, enchondroma, sarcoma, carcinoma

I. Introduction

- Although benign bone and soft tissue lesions in the hand are more common than malignancies, thorough evaluation is necessary prior to treatment.

II. Epidemiology

- Soft tissue tumors of the hand accounts for 15% of all soft tissue tumors.
- Benign lesions are more common than malignancies:
  - Ganglion cysts, epidermal inclusion cysts, and giant cell tumors of tendon sheath (a.k.a. tenosynovial giant cell tumor) are the most common benign soft tissue lesions.
  - Enchondromas, benign cartilage tumors, account for 90% of primary bone tumors of the hand.
  - Epithelioid, synovial sarcoma and chondrosarcoma are the most common malignant soft tissue and bony sarcomas of the hand, respectively.
  - The hand is involved in 0.1% of bony metastases.

III. Diagnosis

- As with other hand pathology, begin with a thorough history and physical examination:
  - Important points to include: Date of symptom onset, mass presence, timeline of progression, character of pain, and neurologic and mechanical symptoms.
  - Intermittent size fluctuations of mass—more likely cystic or vascular, less likely neoplasm.
  - Note mass firmness, mobility, overlying skin changes, local discoloration, neighboring joint range of motion (ROM), neurologic findings, and transillumination.

A. Imaging

- Anteroposterior (AP), lateral, and oblique radiographs generally obtained for all hand masses:
  - Osseous lesions are typically well-demonstrated on plain radiographs.
  - Enchondromas and aneurysmal bone cysts present as lytic, expansile lesions.
  - Soft tissue calcifications, shadows, and local osseous erosion may indicate soft tissue tumor.
- Cross-sectional imaging:
  - MRI is required for diagnosing many tumors, particularly soft tissue tumors. Hyper-intensity on T2-weighted fat-suppressed or short-tau inversion recovery with nodular or mass-like enhancement on T1-weighted postcontrast sequences is concerning for malignancy.
  - CT scan may be useful to further evaluate bony detail, particularly of a presumed osteoid osteoma.
  - Metastatic disease requires appropriate staging studies, including chest CT scan for all sarcomas and whole-body imaging for bone sarcomas.
- Biopsy is generally required for definitive diagnosis of hand tumors. It should be performed by the surgeon planning to definitively treat the tumor:
  - Needle biopsy includes both fine-needle aspiration and core-needle biopsy. These may be image-guided by ultrasound (US) or CT to improve accuracy, but sampling error may still be of concern.
  - Open incisional biopsy should be designed with a subsequent wide resection in mind—the biopsy tract must be excised during final resection. Otherwise commonly used hand incisions (e.g., Bruner's) may not accommodate later digit- or hand-sparing resection.
  - Excisional biopsy may be performed in cases where a benign lesion is suspected with a high degree of certainty, and when excision would not compromise future wide resection if the mass is found to be malignant.

IV. Treatment

A. Benign Lesions

- Benign lesions may often be treated with observation, which may include interval imaging. Diligent monitoring for signs of malignancy is necessary.

1. Soft Tissue Lesions

- Ganglion cysts represent >50% of hand masses:
  - Usually connected to joint by stalk; fluid shifts associated with size fluctuation
  - Most common in dorsal wrist (~65%).
  - Often self-resolving; open or arthroscopic excision is an option for persistent, symptomatic cysts.
- Epidermal inclusion cysts form after subdermal deposition of an epithelial cell, typically in the setting of trauma:
  - Slow-growing, but may erode bone locally.
  - Surgical excision is recommended.
- Lipomas may be safely observed or excised, according to size and symptoms:

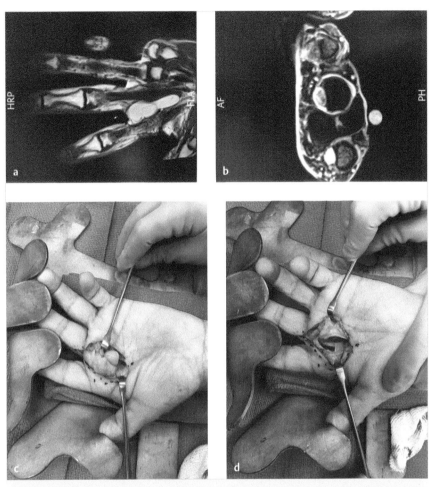

Fig. 23.1 T1 **(a)** and T2 **(b)** noncontrast MRIs of a lipoma of the second web space of the hand with intraoperative images of marginal excision **(c, d)**.

- ○ Well-encapsulated, facilitating excision (▶ Fig. 23.1).
- ○ Atypical lipomatous tumors rarely undergo malignant transformation to liposarcoma.
- Peripheral nerve sheath tumors include schwannomas and neurofibromas:
  - ○ Neurofibromas associated with neurofibromatosis have a higher risk of malignant transformation.
  - ○ If symptoms warrant excision, sacrifice of a nerve may be necessary particularly for neurofibromas—nerve grafting is an option in these cases. Schwannomas may be more easily shelled out from the associated nerve, preserving function.
- Vascular malformations, depending on symptom severity, may be treated with compression garments, sclerotherapy, embolization, or surgical excision in coordination with interventional radiology.

- Tenosynovial giant cell tumor, histologically identical to pigmented villonodular synovitis (PVNS), typically occurs on the palmar hand, but can be found throughout the hand and wrist.
  - Often locally aggressive, warranting excision.
  - Reported recurrence rates as high as approximately 50 to 60%.
- Glomus tumors occur in the subungual region:
  - Arise from the glomus body, a vascular temperature regulator—frequently cause cold hypersensitivity.
  - Surgical excision via nail bed is recommended.
- Periosteal chondromas are rare extramedullary cartilaginous tumors:
  - Typically juxtacortical, may cause scalloping of underlying bone.
  - Recommend resection of adjacent cortex with mass to reduce risk of local recurrence.

2. Benign Bone Lesions

- Benign bone lesions may be observed, if latent, or treated with curettage with or without bone grafting:
  - The proximity of neurovascular structures in the hand may preclude local adjuvant therapy (e.g., cryotherapy, phenol, liquid nitrogen).
- Enchondromas are the most common primary bone tumor of the hand:
  - Lytic, expansile lesion with or without stippled calcifications most often in proximal phalanx (▶ Fig. 23.2).
  - Symptomatic lesions treated with intralesional curettage with or without cement or auto/allograft bone.
  - Recurrence rates after treatment 2 to 15%; malignant transformation of solitary lesions ~1%; regular radiographic surveillance recommended.
  - May be associated with Ollier's disease or Maffucci's syndrome; higher rates of malignant transformation—approximately 25 and 100%, respectively.
- Osteochondromas are exophytic lesions (▶ Fig. 23.3) that may cause mechanical irritation to overlying tendons—can be excised when symptomatic.
- Bizarre parosteal osteochondromatous proliferations (BPOPs) are similarly exophytic and may be excised with periosteum and pseudocapsule to reduce the chance of local recurrence.
- Osteoid osteomas often present as painful lytic lesions, with or without a central nidus:
  - Medical treatment with nonsteroidal anti-inflammatory drugs.
  - If refractory, may pursue surgical excision of lesion and nidus with intralesional curettage or en bloc marginal resection.
  - Radiofrequency ablation, described in other parts of the body, has not been studied in the hand.
- Giant cell tumors of bone typically present as lytic epiphyseal lesions with eccentric osseous involvement:
  - Although benign, may be multifocal and can metastasize to lungs. Chest imaging is required for staging.
  - Treatment is aggressive due to high recurrence rates:
    - Lesions without soft tissue extension—intralesional curettage, with or without local adjuvant therapy, and bone grafting.

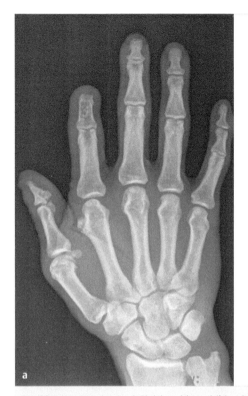
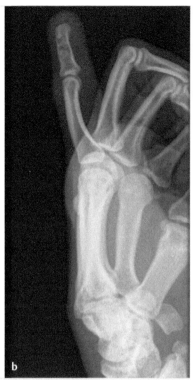

Fig. 23.2 Anteroposterior (AP) **(a)** and lateral **(b)** radiographs of enchondroma of the middle phalanx of the index finger.

- – Lesions with cortical disruption/soft tissue extension—intralesional curettage, with or without local adjuvant therapy, bone grafting versus wide resection and reconstruction.
- ○ Postoperative surveillance for local recurrence and lung metastases required.
- Aneurysmal bone cysts may be treated with intralesional curettage with or without bone grafting initially, with wide resection or even amputation required for large, locally recurrent lesions.

B. Malignant Lesions

- Malignant lesions of the hand, although relatively rare, require close, multidisciplinary care, including appropriate staging studies, adjuvant chemotherapy and radiation therapy when indicated, wide resection, and regular postoperative surveillance.
- Soft tissue sarcomas (STS)
  - ○ Epithelioid sarcoma is the most common STS of the hand:
    - – May present with ulceration and be misdiagnosed as infection which can delay treatment.

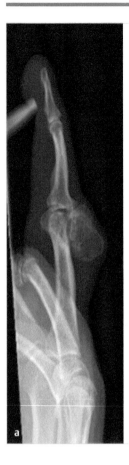
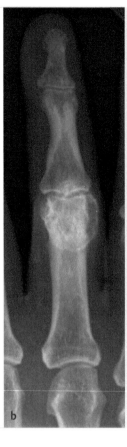

Fig. 23.3 Lateral (a) and anteroposterior (AP) (b) radiographs of an osteochondroma of the middle finger.

– Regional lymph node metastases have been reported in up to 40% of patients, necessitating meticulous examination and possibly sentinel lymph node biopsy (SLNB).

– After wide resection 5-year survival rate approaches 85%.

○ Synovial sarcoma is the second most common STS of the hand:

– Typically arise adjacent to joints or bursae.

– After wide resection/radiation 5-year survival rate approaches 75%.

○ Rhabdomyosarcoma is the most common STS of the hand in children.

• Bony sarcomas

○ Chondrosarcoma typically affects the metacarpals and phalanges:

– X-ray large, lytic, expansile lesion with stippled calcifications.

– Low-grade chondrosarcoma can be difficult to distinguish from enchondroma of the hand. Requires evaluation of pathological, radiological, and clinical findings for diagnosis.

– Chemoradiation and radiation therapy are ineffective.

○ Ewing's sarcoma most often affects adolescents:

– Radiographs may demonstrate a lytic, permeative lesion with cortical destruction/periosteal reaction.

– Adjuvant chemotherapy indicated.

- Local control with wide resection or radiation therapy. Wide surgical resection may have improved rates of local recurrence over radiation in Ewing's sarcoma of extremity.
  - Osteosarcoma rarely occurs in the hand primarily, and can occur secondary to radiation, Paget's disease, or as a metastasis:
    - Characterized by production of osteoid—immature bone.
    - Treat with chemotherapy with wide resection.
- Skin malignancy affecting the hand is most commonly squamous cell carcinoma, followed by basal cell carcinoma and melanoma; wide excision is the mainstay of treatment.
- Metastatic disease to the hand is rare, accounting for 0.1% of osseous metastases:
  - Most frequent primary tumors are lung, breast, and renal.
  - Primary is unknown in 16% of patients presenting with a metastatic hand lesion, necessitating CT of the chest, abdomen, and pelvis and whole-body bone scan, in addition to MRI of the lesion.
  - Life expectancy in patients with hand metastases is 5 to 18 months.

V. Conclusion

- Hand tumors are frequently benign. Thorough evaluation, however, is necessary to guide appropriate treatment. Benign lesions may be treated with observation or marginal/intralesional excision. Malignancies mandate wide resection and multidisciplinary oncologic care.

Suggested Readings

Baumhoer D, Jundt G. Tumours of the hand: a review on histology of bone malignancies. J Hand Surg Eur Vol. 2010; 35(5):354–361

Hayden RJ, Sullivan LG, Jebson PJ. The hand in metastatic disease and acral manifestations of paraneoplastic syndromes. Hand Clin. 2004; 20(3):335–343, vii

Hsu CS, Hentz VR, Yao J. Tumours of the hand. Lancet Oncol. 2007; 8(2):157–166

Payne WT, Merrell G. Benign bony and soft tissue tumors of the hand. J Hand Surg Am. 2010; 35(11):1901–1910

Puhaindran ME, Rohde RS, Chou J, Morris CD, Athanasian EA. Clinical outcomes for patients with soft tissue sarcoma of the hand. Cancer. 2011; 117(1):175–179

24 Congenital Conditions of the Upper Extremity and Hand

Danielle A. Hogarth and Joshua M. Abzug

Abstract

Congenital conditions affecting the upper extremity are observed in 1 in every 600 to 700 live births. These conditions derive from failure of upper limb development during gestation. Surgical intervention is often warranted to correct functional limitations and minimize aesthetic differences for both the child and their family. Conditions like syndactyly, polydactyly, thumb hypoplasia, and constriction band syndrome often undergo surgical intervention due to the limited potential complications but substantial functional and aesthetic benefits. Therapy and continual observation may be a more ideal treatment strategy for other conditions such as radial longitudinal deficiency or type I polydactyly if it does not infringe on prehension function or if the patient has been able to compensate accordingly. Should surgical intervention be elected, it typically is performed within the first 2 years of age or soon after functional limitations are present. Corrective surgeries of congenital conditions affecting the hand aim to provide bilateral symmetry, adequate prehension, and regain functional upper extremity ability for children while minimizing aesthetic differences, where possible.

Keywords: Congenital conditions, hand, upper extremity, embryology, polydactyly, syndactyly, radial longitudinal deficiency, thumb hypoplasia, synostosis

I. Embryology

- Congenital hand differences vary in their functional and aesthetic implications.
- Rapid limb bud development occurs between weeks 4 and 8 of fetal gestation.[1,2]
- Fibroblast growth factors regulate sonic hedgehog (SHH) gene which is responsible for proper limb structures development from the limb bud.
- Understanding the affected axis can provide insight on the underlying etiology of the abnormality:
  - Apical ectodermal ridge (AER): Regulates longitudinal growth.[2]
  - Zone of polarizing activity (ZPA): Regulates development of ulnar and radial structures and other growth about the anteroposterior axis.[2]
  - Wnt signaling pathway: Determines development of dorsal and ventral structures.[2]

II. Polydactyly

A. Incidence

- 1 per 300 to 1 per 3,000 births.
- More common in African–American population than Caucasian.
- Type IV is the most common (43%) followed by Type II (15%).

B. Etiology/Genetics

- Typically, unilateral and random.
- Exact etiology is not well known.

C. Classification

- Duplication of digits.
- Preaxial: Thumb duplication (Wassel classification; ▶ Fig. 24.1 and ▶ Table 24.1).
- Central: Duplication at the midline.
- Postaxial: Small finger duplication (▶ Fig. 24.2):
  ○ Type A: Well-formed digit articulating with the fifth metacarpal.
  ○ Type B: Skin tag or a rudimentary pedunculated digit (▶ Fig. 24.2).[3]

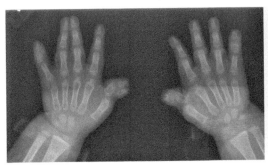

Fig. 24.1 Radiograph of bilateral preaxial polydactyly: Left thumb Wassel Type II, right thumb Wassel Type I. (Courtesy of Joshua M. Abzug, MD)

Table 24.1 Wassel classification of preaxial polydactyly

Type I	Bifid distal phalanx with a common epiphysis which articulates with a normal proximal phalanx typically seen with two distinct nails with a groove between them
Type II	Complete duplication of distal phalanx—each phalanx has its own epiphysis which articulates with the normal proximal phalanx
Type III	Duplicated distal phalanx with a bifurcated proximal phalanx that typically diverge from the longitudinal axis
Type IV	Complete duplication of proximal phalanx—each phalanx has its own epiphysis or a common epiphysis that articulates with a normal metacarpal or a slightly widened metacarpal to accommodate both proximal phalanges
Type V	Bifurcated first metacarpal—each head of the bifurcation articulates with a duplicated proximal phalanx that has its own epiphysis
Type VI	Complete duplication of the metacarpal and entire first digit
Type VII	Triphalangeal thumb or elements of a triphalangeal thumb accompanying by a normal thumb

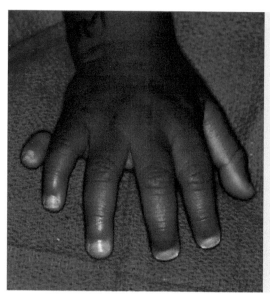

Fig. 24.2 Clinical photograph of a Type B postaxial polydactyly. (Courtesy of Joshua M. Abzug, MD)

D. Treatment

1. Surgical Treatment

- Preaxial: Goal is to reconstruct a thumb that attains bilateral symmetry while preserving pinch function:
  - Types I, II, and III: Bilhaut–Cloquet procedure involves removing central tissue and combining both digits into one.
  - Types III and IV: Type 2 combination technique preserves skeleton and nail of one component and augment with soft tissue from other digit; ablation of lesser digit.
  - Types V, VI, and VIII: Type 3 combination technique involves segmental digital transfer.
- Central: Goal is to remove extra digit in order to prevent angular growth deformities.
  - Osteotomy and ligamentous reconstructions.
- Postaxial: Goal is typically to remove lesser digit:
  - Type A: Reconstruction with Type 2 combination technique preserves radial digit, radial collateral ligaments, and muscular structures.
  - Type B: Suture ligation—tie off in nursery or amputate before age 1, essentially inducing avascular necrosis to the rudimentary digit.

III. Syndactyly

A. Incidence

- Seen in 1 per 2,000 to 3,000 live births.[1,4,5]
- More prevalent in males than in females.

B. Etiology/Genetics

- Autosomal dominant.
- Syndactyly occurs secondary to failure of apoptotic mechanisms that typically create webspaces between digits between weeks 6 and 8 of gestation.[6]
- Disturbed Wnt signaling and gap junction protein function lead to syndactyly.[2]
- Associated conditions:
  - Constriction band syndrome.
  - Poland's syndrome.
  - Apert syndrome.
  - Carpenter's syndrome.

C. Classification

- Connection of adjacent digits (▶ Fig. 24.3).
- Described by degree of connection:
  - Complete: Connected the full length of the digits (▶ Fig. 24.3a).
  - Incomplete: Proximal connection of adjacent fingers (▶ Fig. 24.3b).
- Described by type of connected tissue:
  - Simple: Connected by skin only.
  - Complex: Skeletal, muscular, and cutaneous fusion of adjacent digits.
- Synechia: Unique condition where all digits (index to small) are completely connected as well as a connection between the nail plates.

D. Treatment

- Hand function and aesthetic preference are the primary determinants of whether surgical intervention is warranted.

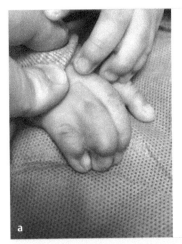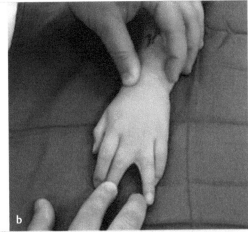

Fig. 24.3 Clinical photographs of **(a)** a complete long-ring-small syndactyly status post separation of the tips of the ring and small fingers and **(b)** an incomplete long-ring syndactyly. (Courtesy of Joshua M. Abzug, MD)

1. Nonoperative Management

- Simple, incomplete cases can be addressed according to patient and family's preference as these presentations do not substantially limit hand function.

2. Surgical Treatment

- Digit release
  - Complete, complex syndactyly with nail involvement (flag and pennant technique—use skin from pulp of each digit to reconstruct the lateral nail fold).
    - Interdigitating zigzag flaps to avoid longitudinal scarring.
  - Partial syndactyly can be treated with skin flaps with possible application of skin grafts or skin graft alternatives:
    - Island flaps.
    - Three-square flap.
  - Full-thickness skin grafts are standard to obtain skin coverage following digital separation.

E. Complications

- Recurrent web creep or resyndactylization is the most common complication following digital release.

IV. Thumb Hypoplasia

A. Incidence

- 1 per 30,000 live births.[7]

B. Etiology/Genetics

- Exact etiology is not well known.[8]
- On the radial longitudinal deficiency spectrum; therefore, associated organ system conditions may be affected as well.[8]
  - VACTERAL (vertebral defects, anal atresia, cardiac defects, tracheo-esophageal fistula, renal anomalies, and limb abnormalities).
  - Holt—Oram syndrome.
  - Thrombocytopenia absent radius (TAR).
  - Fanconi anemia.

C. Classification

- Congenital underdevelopment of the thumb[8,9] (▶ Fig. 24.4 and ▶ Table 24.2).

D. Treatment

1. Nonoperative Management

- Type I: Observation is warranted to ensure that thumb and hand function are not substantially limited.

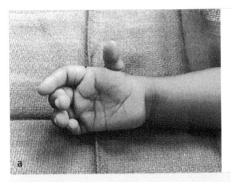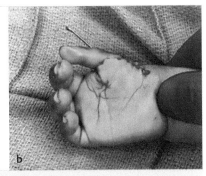

Fig. 24.4 Clinical photograph of a Type IIIB hypoplastic thumb: (a) preoperative and (b) status post index finger pollicization. Note the unstable thumb carpometacarpal joint preoperatively. (Courtesy of Joshua M. Abzug, MD)

Table 24.2 Blauth classification of hypoplastic thumb

Type I	Minor hypoplasia—slightly decreased thumb size
Type II	Narrowed first webspace, hypoplastic thenar musculature, unstable MCP joint
Type III	A: Stable CMC joint; extrinsic muscle abnormalities B: Unstable CMC joint; extrinsic muscle abnormalities
Type IV	Pouce flottant or floating thumb
Type V	Complete absence of thumb

Abbreviations: CMC, carpometacarpal; MCP, metacarpophalangeal.

2. Surgical Treatment

- Stability of carpometacarpal (CMC) joint dictates whether reconstruction or pollicization procedures are indicated:[8,10]
  - Type II: Oppensplasty to release the first webspace and increase range of motion.[10,11]
  - Type IIIA: Thumb reconstruction.
  - Types IIIB, V, and VI: Ablation of the existing digit with subsequent pollicization procedure[11,12] (▶ Fig. 24.4).

V. Radioulnar Synostosis

A. Incidence

- Very rare congenital disorder with only 350 cases reported in the literature.[13]
- Affects males more than females.

B. Etiology/Genetics

- Failure of differentiation of the cartilaginous precursors into the radius and ulna in week 7 of gestation.

- One out of five cases positive with family history: Autosomal dominant inherence pattern.
- Associated conditions in 30% of cases:
  - Apert syndrome
  - Carpenter's syndrome
  - Arthrogryposis
  - Mandibulofacial dysostosis
  - Klinefelter's syndrome
  - Sex chromosome abnormalities

C. Classification

- Bony bridge between the proximal radius and ulna determined by radiographic findings.
- Presentation is typically delayed until late childhood when forearm rotation is more incorporated into daily life (e.g., child catching a ball, holding a pencil) (▶ Table 24.3).

D. Treatment

1. Nonoperative Management

- Observation for asymptomatic and unilateral cases where lack of forearm rotation has been adequately compensated for (excessive shoulder rotation).

2. Surgical Treatment

- Synostosis excision with soft tissue interposition: Restores active forearm rotation.
- Forearm derotational osteotomy: Places the forearm in a more functional resting position.

E. Complications

- Poor surgical outcomes due to poorly or underdeveloped surrounding structures, neurovascular compromise, and recurrence of the synostosis.
  - Recurrence of synostosis: Guaranteed recurrence without interposition of vascularized fascio-fat graft to maintain separation.
  - Recurrence of malrotation: Casting after derotational osteotomy may be associated with loss of correction; can be regained with therapy focused on active range of motion.

Table 24.3 Cleary classification of radioulnar synostosis

Type 1	No osseous synostosis	No radial head dislocation
Type 2	Osseous synostosis	No radial head dislocation
Type 3	Long osseous synostosis	Hypoplastic radial head, posterior dislocation
Type 4	Short osseous synostosis	Radial head deformation, anterior dislocation

- Compartment syndrome: Associated with large rotational corrections; has been limited with prophylactic forearm fasciotomies.
- Neurologic deficit: Most resolve within 3 months:
  - Posterior interosseous nerve (PIN) palsy.
  - Anterior interosseous nerve (AIN) palsy.
  - Radial nerve palsy.

VI. Radial Longitudinal Deformity

A. Incidence

- Reported incidence from 1 in 30,000 to 1 in 100,000 live births.[14,15,16,17]

B. Etiology/Genetics

- Sonic hedgehog gene influence:
  - Caused by the reduction of fibroblast growth factors that are typically responsible for development of limb along radial-ulnar/anteroposterior axis occurring between weeks 4 and 7 of gestation.[18,19]
  - The reduced function of fibroblast growth factors limits outgrowth of the radius while the zone of polarized activity (ZPA) remains intact, thus causing a radial deficiency while ulnar structures continue to typically develop.[19]
- Associated organ abnormalities:
  - Holt-Oram syndrome: An autosomal dominant condition that presents with cardiac septal defects and variable phenotypes of radial hypoplasia.
  - Fanconi anemia: A pancytopenia that results in complete bone marrow destruction at approximately 7 years of age.
  - TAR syndrome: A pathognomonic phenotype with absent radii and broad, flat thumbs.
  - Diamond Blackfan syndrome: A very rare condition, but also has associated cardiac and hematologic disorders, with anemia as the most common presentation; inheritance is most often autosomal dominant.
  - VACTERL syndrome: Vertebral anomalies, anal atresia, cardiac abnormalities, tracheoesophageal fistula, renal agenesis, and limb defects commonly associated with radial longitudinal deficiency (RLD).

C. Classification

- Improper development of the radius and associated radial structures (▶ Table 24.4 and ▶ Fig. 24.5).

Table 24.4 Bayne and Klug classification of radial longitudinal deficiency

Type 1	Deficient distal radial epiphysis
Type 2	Deficient distal and proximal radial epiphyses
Type 3	Present proximally (partial aplasia)
Type 4	Completely absent radius

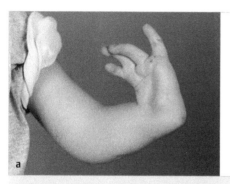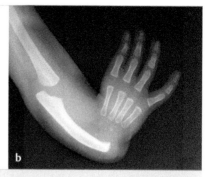

Fig. 24.5 (a) Clinical photograph and (b) radiograph of a child with Type 4 radial longitudinal deficiency. Note the complete absence of the radius and the thumb. (Courtesy of Joshua M. Abzug, MD)

D. Treatment

1. Nonoperative Management

- Mild presentations: Passive stretching and serial splinting/casting to straighten out bowing of extremity and to realign carpus with ulna while maintaining the range of motion of the wrist.[16]
- Observation:
  - Older patients can function with compensatory mechanisms.
  - Patients with elbow extension contracture who rely on radial deviation to reach midline and perform activities of daily living (ADLs).

2. Surgical Treatment

- Wrist realignment:
  - Centralization: Arthroplasty technique to realign the carpus with the ulna via transverse ulnar incision.[20]
  - Radialization: Straightening the wrist while transferring flexor carpi radialis and extensor carpi radialis tendons to the ulnar side.[21]
- Ulnocarpal arthrodesis: Performed in cases with greater than 45 degrees of radial angulation.
- Ulnar lengthening: To increase forearm length simultaneously correcting radial deviation.[22]

VII. Trigger Thumb (Stenosing Tenosynovitis of the Flexor Pollicis Longus Tendon)

A. Incidence

- Acquired as early as first 2 months of life—incidence is 3 per 1,000 live births.[23,24]
- One in four cases present with bilateral trigger thumb.[25]
- Nearly equal distribution between females (60%) and males (40%).[22]

B. Etiology/Genetics

- Etiology is not well known as to whether its congenital or acquired condition.[26]

C. Classification

- Fixed flexion of the thumb interphalangeal (IP) joint caused by inflammation of the flexor tendon sheath.
- Palpable nodule present at the annular pulley (A-1) region, also known as Notta's nodule.[23]

D. Treatment

- Nonoperative management should be attempted before surgery is considered.
- About 30 to 60% of cases can resolve spontaneously after a bout of observation.[27]

1. Nonoperative Management

- Passive extension splinting, 65% showed full thumb motion after contiguous splinting.[28]
- Observation with intermittent extension splinting.

2. Surgical Treatment

- A-1 pulley release is the most commonly performed procedure:
  - Small incision over thumb metacarpophalangeal (MCP) flexion crease, extending over the A-1 pulley region.
  - Sharp dissection of the A-1 pulley.
  - Identify Notta's nodule in flexor pollicis longus (FPL) tendon.
  - Under direct vision during passive IP extension ensure there is smooth FPL tendon gliding.
- Resolution rate is 92.3% after A-1 pulley release.[27]

VIII. Symbrachydactyly

A. Incidence

- Congenital hand malformation condition—transverse deficiency.
- Approximately 0.6 per 10,000 live births.[29]
- Typically, isolated presentation, but can be associated with other congenital conditions such as Poland's syndrome.
- Often unilateral presentation.

B. Etiology/Genetics

- Exact etiology is not well known.
- Hypothesized that vascular dysgenesis of the subclavian artery supply during fetal development is the leading cause.

- Transverse deficiency caused by disruption of the apical ectodermal ridge (AER) of the limb bud within the first 4 to 6 weeks of gestation resulting in abnormal proximal-distal development.

C. Classification

- Characterized by failure of formation of fingers as well as presence of rudimentary nubbins with nail plate, bone, and cartilage.[29]
- Central digits (third and fourth) are most commonly affected (▶ Fig. 24.6, ▶ Fig. 24.7, and ▶ Table 24.5).

D. Treatment

- Goals are to maximize function, normalize appearance, and help the patient and family to accept the differences should "normal" is not able to be achieved.
- Treatment protocols dictated by clinical and radiological findings, relative ability of the patient to perform ADLs, hand appearance, and thumb function.

1. Nonoperative Management

- Therapy: Goal is to master ADLs while gaining functional independence with the affected side (▶ Fig. 24.6 and ▶ Fig. 24.7).
- Orthotics/prosthetics: Can help with achieving a more normal appearance; however, they are not functional as the sensation is missing.
  - Not typically recommended, rather gaining independence and mastering ADLs are suggested.
- Regular treatment with an occupational therapist may be recommended to assist patients with mastering ADLs.

2. Surgical Treatment

- Surgical treatment categorized by the specific aspect of the condition.
- Syndactyly and web contracture: Syndactyly release and web deepening.
- Brachydactyly and digit instability: Phalanx transfers or distraction lengthening.

IX. Constriction Band Syndrome

A. Incidence

- Area most often affected is distal to the wrist, particularly at the hands/fingers.
- Reported incidence from 1 per 1,200 to 1 per 15,000 live births.[30,31,32]

B. Etiology/Genetics

- Exact etiology is unknown, but primarily theories include intrinsic or extrinsic theory:[30]
  - Streeter's intrinsic theory: An endogenous defect in germ plasm differentiation causes a necrotic limb and fibrous band formation.

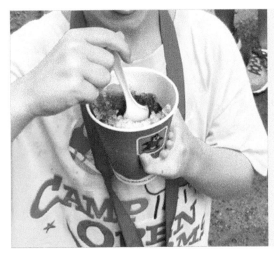

Fig. 24.6 Clinical photograph of a child with Type II symbrachydactyly. Note the ability to grasp between the thumb and small finger. (Courtesy of Joshua M. Abzug, MD)

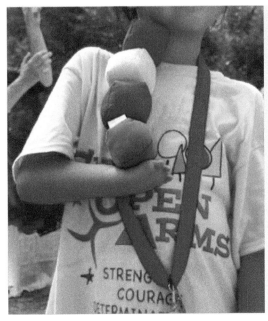

Fig. 24.7 Clinical photograph of a child with Type IV symbrachydactyly. (Courtesy of Joshua M. Abzug, MD)

- ○ Torpin's extrinsic theory: Ruptured or disrupted amnion releases fibrous membranous strands that surround developing limb reducing blood supply to the distal portion ultimately inhibiting proper development and causing autoamputation.
- Prematurity (less than 37 weeks), low birth weight (less than 2,500 g), maternal illness or trauma, and maternal drug exposure have been noted as prenatal risk factors.[30]
- Sporadic hereditary pattern.

Table 24.5 Foucher classification of symbrachydactyly

Type I: Short finger type	All bones and digits present, brachydactyly and syndactyly
Type II: Cleft hand type	A: At least two fingers, normal thumb, hypoplastic fingers B: Functional border digits, variable central nubbins C: Spoon hand, thumb conjoined with hypoplastic ulnar digits
Type III: Monodactyly type	A: Monodactyly with normal thumb development B: Monodactyly with hypoplastic and/or unstable thumb
Type IV: Peromelic type	A: Peromelic, wrist mobility B: Peromelic, no wrist mobility

Table 24.6 Patterson classification of constriction band syndrome

Type I	Simple constriction ring
Type II	Deformity distal to ring (hypoplasia, lymphedema)
Type III	Fusions distally (syndactyly, acrosyndactyly)
Type IV	Amputation, loss of limb distal to ring

C. Classification

- Intrauterine diagnosis can be made via ultrasound by the end of the first trimester (▶ Table 24.6).

D. Treatment

- Goal is to alleviate distal deformity while regaining maximal hand function.
- Interference with circulation or lymphatic drainage is the primary reason for pursuing operative measures.

E. Nonoperative Management

- Observation
  - Indicated for Type I.

F. Surgical Treatment[30]

- Excision or release of constriction band (indicated for Type I).
- Circumferential Z-plasties (indicated for Type II).
- Surgical release of syndactyly (indicated for Type III).
- Reconstruction of involved digits (indicated for Type IV).

X. Camptodactyly

A. Incidence

- More often bilateral presentations.
- Most commonly affects little finger.

Table 24.7 Benson classification of camptodactyly

Type I	Isolated contracture of little finger PIP (most common form), presents in infancy
Type II	• Isolated contracture of little finger PIP, presents in adolescents • Due to abnormal lumbrical insertion or flexor digitorum superficialis origin or insertion
Type III	Severe contractures, multiple digits involved, presents at birth
Kirner's deformity	• Specific deformity of small finger DIP with volar-radial curvature • Often bilateral • Often affects preadolescent girls

Abbreviations: DIP, distal interphalangeal; PIP, proximal interphalangeal.

B. Etiology/Genetics

• May be associated with more widespread developmental dysmorphology syndromes.

C. Classification

• Congenital digital flexion contracture of proximal interphalangeal (PIP) joint (▶ Table 24.7).

D. Treatment

1. Nonoperative Management

• Passive stretching, splinting using orthoses.
  ○ Indicated for most cases (angulation less than 30 degrees).
• Earlier intervention when possible.

2. Surgical Treatment

• Flexor digitorum superficialis tenotomy with or without a tendon transfer.[33]
  ○ Indicated for cases of progressive deformity that causes a functional impairment after unsuccessful attempts with orthosis use.
• Osteotomy versus arthrodesis.[33]
  ○ Indicated for severely fixed deformities.

XI. Clinodactyly

A. Classification

• Radial deviation of small finger due to an abnormal middle phalanx[34] (▶ Table 24.8).

B. Treatment

• Rarely painful or functionally limiting.
• Surgical management only beneficial if the patient has serious functional limitations of the hand.[34]

Table 24.8 Classification of clinodactyly

Type I	Minor angulation with normal length
Type II	Minor angulation with short length
Type III	Significant angulation and delta phalanx (c-shaped epiphysis and longitudinal bracketed diaphysis)

1. Nonoperative Management

- Observation: Ensure that the digit does not develop more severe angulation or impede on hand function with continued longitudinal growth.

2. Surgical Treatment

- Osteotomy: Removing extra bone to straighten the affected phalanx.
- Physiolysis with fat transposition: Correction of the unaffected side allowing for restoration of symmetrical, longitudinal growth of the middle phalanx.[35]

XII. Madelung's Deformity

A. Etiology/Genetics

- Commonly observed in adolescent (ages 8–13) females.
- Most cases are a symptomatic until adolescent age as the magnitude of the deformity worsens with accelerated skeletal growth.[36]
- Exact etiology is unknown, but there is a proposed genetic component (autosomal dominant):
  - Associated with Leri-Weill dyschondrosteosis (a mesomelic form of dwarfism).

B. Classification

- Premature, partial arrest of the distal radial physis causing radial bowing, ulnar carpal impaction, and volar subluxation of the radius (▶ Fig. 24.8).
- Typically bilateral presentation.

C. Treatment

1. Nonoperative Management

- Observation: Regular radiographs to ensure radial bowing and carpal impaction do not worsen significantly.
- Restricted activity: Refrain from engaging in upper extremity weight-bearing activities such as push-ups and participating in gymnastics until pain is relieved.

2. Surgical Treatment

- Physiolysis with release of Vickers ligament: Indicated for skeletally immature patients with wrist pain and decreased range of motion of the wrist.[37]

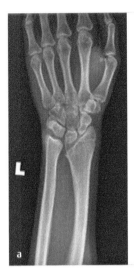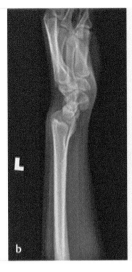

Fig. 24.8 Radiographs of a Madelung's deformity. **(a)** Posteroanterior (PA) view and **(b)** lateral view. (Courtesy of Joshua M. Abzug, MD)

- Bilateral radial and ulnar epiphysiodesis: Indicated for patients with good range of motion of the wrist with nearly closed growth plates.[37]
- Radial corrective osteotomy: Indicated for patients with nearly or fully closed growth plates to alleviate wrist pain, limited range of motion, and correct bowing deformity.[37]

References

[1] Kozin SH. Syndactyly. J Hand Surg Am. 2001; 1(1):1–13
[2] Al-Qattan MM, Kozin SH. Update on embryology of the upper limb. J Hand Surg Am. 2013; 38(9):1835–1844
[3] Abzug JM, Kozin SH. Treatment of postaxial polydactyly type B. J Hand Surg Am. 2013; 38(6):1223–1225
[4] Tonkin MA. Failure of differentiation part I: Syndactyly. Hand Clin. 2009; 25(2):171–193
[5] Flatt AE. Webbed fingers. Proc Bayl Univ Med Cent. 2005; 18(1):26–37
[6] Wilkie AO, Patey SJ, Kan SH, van den Ouweland AM, Hamel BC. FGFs, their receptors, and human limb malformations: clinical and molecular correlations. Am J Med Genet. 2002; 112(3):266–278
[7] Ekblom AG, Laurell T, Arner M. Epidemiology of congenital upper limb anomalies in 562 children born in 1997 to 2007: a total population study from Stockholm, Sweden. J Hand Surg Am. 2010; 35(11):1742–1754
[8] Soldado F, Zlotolow DA, Kozin SH. Thumb hypoplasia. J Hand Surg Am. 2013; 38(7):1435–1444
[9] Blauth W, Schneider-Sickert F, eds. Congenital Deformities of the Hand. An Atlas of Their Surgical Treatment. Berlin, Germany: Spinger; 1982
[10] Little KJ, Cornwall R. Congenital anomalies of the hand—principles of management. Orthop Clin North Am. 2016; 47(1):153–168
[11] Sullivan MA, Adkinson JM. Congenital hand differences. Plast Surg Nurs. 2016; 36(2):84–89
[12] Tsai J. Congenital radioulnar synostosis. Radiol Case Rep. 2017; 12(3):552–554
[13] Geck MJ, Dorey F, Lawrence JF, Johnson MK. Congenital radius deficiency: radiographic outcome and survivorship analysis. J Hand Surg Am. 1999; 24(6):1132–1144
[14] Maschke SD, Seitz W, Lawton J. Radial longitudinal deficiency. J Am Acad Orthop Surg. 2007; 15(1):41–52
[15] Kotwal PP, Varshney MK, Soral A. Comparison of surgical treatment and nonoperative management for radial longitudinal deficiency. J Hand Surg Eur Vol. 2012; 37(2):161–169
[16] Urban MA, Osterman AL. Management of radial dysplasia. Hand Clin. 1990; 6(4):589–605
[17] Colen DL, Lin IC, Levin LS, Chang B. Radial longitudinal deficiency: recent developments, controversies, and an evidence-based guide to treatment. J Hand Surg Am. 2017; 42(7):546–563
[18] Bauer AS, Bednar MS, James MA. Disruption of the radial/ulnar axis: congenital longitudinal deficiencies. J Hand Surg Am. 2013; 38(11):2293–2302, quiz 2302

[19] Manske PR, McCarroll HR, Jr, Swanson K. Centralization of the radial club hand: an ulnar surgical approach. J Hand Surg Am. 1981; 6(5):423–433

[20] Buck-Gramcko D. Radialization as a new treatment for radial club hand. J Hand Surg Am. 1985; 10(6 Pt 2):964–968

[21] Abzug JM, Kozin SH. Radial longitudinal deficiency. J Hand Surg Am. 2014; 39(6):1180–1182

[22] Weilby A. Trigger finger. Incidence in children and adults and the possibility of a predisposition in certain age groups. Acta Orthop Scand. 1970; 41(4):419–427

[23] Rodgers WB, Waters PM. Incidence of trigger digits in newborns. J Hand Surg Am. 1994; 19(3):364–368

[24] Steenwerckx A, De Smet L, Fabry G. Congenital trigger digit. J Hand Surg Am. 1996; 21(5):909–911

[25] Herdem M, Bayram H, Toğrul E, Sarpel Y. Clinical analysis of the trigger thumb of childhood. Turk J Pediatr. 2003; 45(3):237–239

[26] Baek GH, Kim JH, Chung MS, Kang SB, Lee YH, Gong HS. The natural history of pediatric trigger thumb. J Bone Joint Surg Am. 2008; 90(5):980–985

[27] Womack ME, Ryan JC, Shillingford-Cole V, Speicher S, Hogue GD. Treatment of paediatric trigger finger: a systematic review and treatment algorithm. J Child Orthop. 2018; 12(3):209–217

[28] Farr S, Grill F, Ganger R, Girsch W. Open surgery versus nonoperative treatments for paediatric trigger thumb: a systematic review. J Hand Surg Eur Vol. 2014; 39(7):719–726

[29] Goodell PB, Bauer AS, Sierra FJ, James MA. Symbrachydactyly. Hand (N Y). 2016; 11(3):262–270

[30] Kawamura K, Chung KC. Constriction band syndrome. Hand Clin. 2009; 25(2):257–264

[31] Baker CJ, Rudolph AJ. Congenital ring constrictions and intrauterine amputations. Am J Dis Child. 1971; 121 (5):393–400

[32] Seeds JW, Cefalo RC, Herbert WN. Amniotic band syndrome. Am J Obstet Gynecol. 1982; 144(3):243–248

[33] Wall LB, Ezaki M, Goldfarb CA. Camptodactyly treatment for the lesser digits. J Hand Surg Am. 2018; 43 (9):874.e1–874.e4

[34] Goldfarb CA. Congenital hand differences. J Hand Surg Am. 2009; 34(7):1351–1356

[35] El Sayed L, Salon A, Glorion C, Guero S. Physiolysis for correction of clinodactyly with delta phalanx: early improvement. Hand Surg Rehabil. 2019; 38(2):125–128

[36] Ghatan AC, Hanel DP. Madelung deformity. J Am Acad Orthop Surg. 2013; 21(6):372–382

[37] Saffar P, Badina A. Treatment of Madelung's deformity. Chir Main. 2015; 34(6):279–285

25 Fractures of the Pediatric Hand

James S. Lin and Julie B. Samora

Abstract

Hand fractures are common injuries in children and adolescents. There are unique management considerations in skeletally immature patients. Clinical examination may be difficult in anxious children with varying capacities to communicate. Open physes and incomplete carpal ossification may make fracture identification challenging on radiographs. Smaller anatomy also contributes to the challenges in diagnosis and treatment. Fortunately, the robust periosteum and skeletal healing potential of children usually allow for excellent outcomes oftentimes without need for operative intervention. However, the robust healing potential also necessitates prompt identification and management of pediatric hand fractures to prevent skeletal deformities in those injuries that require more than conservative intervention. Furthermore, adherence to rehabilitation and immobilization protocols may also be a concern for children. In this section, common pediatric hand fracture patterns and management principles are reviewed.

Keywords: Pediatrics, children, hand fractures, finger fractures

I. Extra-octave Fractures

A. Background

- Juxta-epiphyseal Salter-Harris type II fracture.
- Transverse fracture through the proximal phalanx physis or metaphysis of the small digit.
- Most common fracture pattern of the proximal phalanx in children.[1]

B. Presentation

- Injured digit is typically abducted and angulated (▶ Fig. 25.1):
  - Usually in ulnar deviation.[2]

C. Mechanism of Injury

- Forced abduction of the small finger from direct impact or sporting activities.

D. Treatment

1. Closed Reduction and Immobilization + /– Kirschner-Wire (K-Wire) Fixation

- Indications
  - Most fractures can be treated with closed reduction and casting or splinting:
    - Proximity of the fracture to the physis allows for significant remodeling.[3]
  - Pin fixation may be required to hold reduction if unstable.

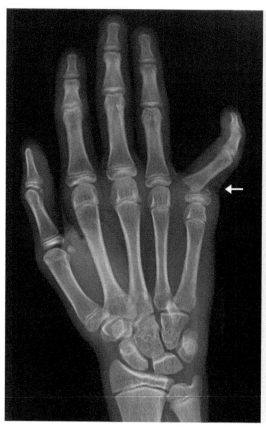

Fig. 25.1 Extra-octave fracture of right hand of a 12-year-old male sustained when a football had direct impact of the small finger. Note the abduction deformity of the injured small digit.

- Techniques
  - Reduction may be aided by the "pencil technique"
    - Involves placing a pencil (or other long thin instrument such as a freer elevator) deep within the fourth web space.
    - Helps control the proximal segment of the fracture and provide a lever arm.
    - Distal finger can be directed radially over the lever arm.[4]
  - Immobilization for 3 weeks with splinting or casting typically required.
  - Buddy taping after immobilization until full range of motion is achieved (▶ Fig. 25.2).

2. Open Reduction and Immobilization + /– K-Wire Fixation

- Indications
  - Fractures unable to be close reduced, possibly due to:
    - Comminution
    - Soft tissue entrapment (i.e., flexor tendons)
    - Associated collateral ligament disruption

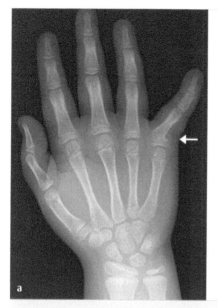 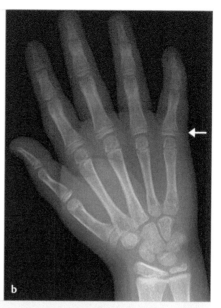

Fig. 25.2 Extra-octave fracture noted on the plain anteroposterior (AP) radiographs of a 6-year-old girl following a trampoline injury **(a)**. 11 days post reduction, with radiographic evidence of healing already present **(b)**.

II. Phalangeal Neck Fractures

A. Background

- Predominantly pediatric injuries.[4]

B. Presentation

- Affected interphalangeal joint is typically hyperextended.
- Flexion is blocked due to obliteration of the subcondylar fossa.[3]
- Fractures usually dorsally displaced and highly unstable:
  ○ Complication rates higher than all other pediatric hand fractures.[5,6,7]

C. Mechanism of Injury

- Commonly when digit is entrapped in a closing door, and the child reflexively withdraws his or her hand.
  ○ This imposes a rotational force that displaces the distal fragment.
- Sports and falls are also common etiologies.[8]

D. Evaluation Considerations

- Three radiographic views (anteroposterior [AP], lateral, and oblique).
- Assess malrotation and radial/ulnar deviation on clinical examination.

E. Classification

- Al-Qattan classification system based on displacement and bony contact (▶ Fig. 25.3):[9]
  - Type I
    - Nondisplaced
    - Relatively stable
  - Type II
    - Any degree of displacement
    - Bone-to-bone contact at the fracture site remains
    - Unstable fractures
  - Type III
    - Displaced
    - Bony apposition at the fracture site is lost entirely.[9]
- Types II and III can both be subclassified into four subtypes based on fracture configuration and rotation/location of the phalangeal head, respectively.[10]

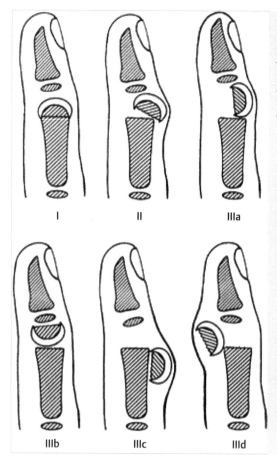

Fig. 25.3 Classification of phalangeal neck fractures based on displacement and bony contact. Used, with permission, from: Al-Qattan MM. Phalangeal neck fractures in children: classification and outcome in 66 cases. J Hand Surg Br. 2001;26 (2):112–121.

F. Treatment

- Splinting or casting alone:
  - Indications
    - Completely nondisplaced (type I) fractures.[9]
  - Close (weekly) radiographic follow-up is required to detect late displacement.
- Closed reduction and percutaneous pin fixation
  - Indications
    - Most phalangeal neck fractures are displaced and therefore treated operatively.
    - Anatomic reduction is imperative for good functional outcomes.
    - Pin fixation usually required to prevent redisplacement.[8,9,11]
    - Type IIa (transverse fracture line at the phalangeal neck) most common.[10]
  - Techniques
    - Closed reduction attempted in the operating room.
    - Subsequent K-wire fixation to maintain the reduction once confirmed by fluoroscopy (▶ Fig. 25.4).
    - Patient should then be cast immobilized until pin removal at approximately 4 weeks; motion can be initiated at this point.
- Percutaneous reduction (osteoclasis technique) and pin fixation.
  - Indications.
    - Above indications, if closed reduction is inadequate, or for subacute fractures.
  - Use a K-wire to manipulate the fracture fragment to its anatomic position.[8,10,12,13]
- Open reduction and pin fixation:
  - Indications.
    - Above indications and if closed and percutaneous reduction is inadequate.
    - Sometimes required for type III fractures.
  - Care should be taken to protect collateral ligament attachments.
    - Preserve collateral ligaments to preserve blood supply.
    - Risk of avascular necrosis becomes greater with an open technique.[8,14]

G. Complications

1. Osteonecrosis

- High rates with type III fractures.[10,15]

2. Persistent Deformity, Malunion, Nonunion

- Remodeling potential is limited due to the great distance from the phalangeal neck to the physis at the proximal phalangeal metaphysis.[7,9,10]

3. Malunions

- Established (as opposed to incipient[12]) malunions.
- Treatment.
- Some propose delaying surgical reconstruction to wait for fracture remodeling if:
  - Malunion occurs only in the sagittal plane.
  - The adjacent joint is congruent.
  - Significant growth potential remains.
  - Family is willing to wait.[16]

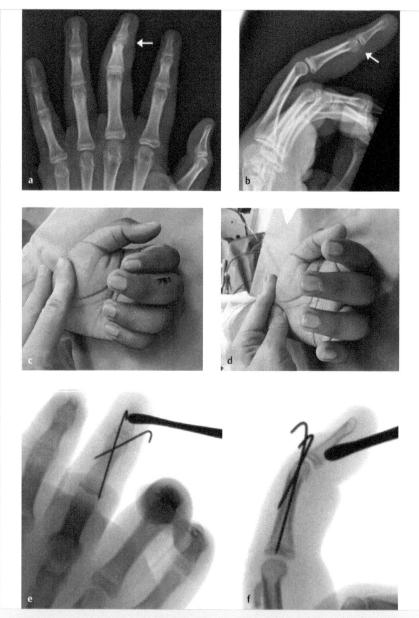

Fig. 25.4 Anteroposterior (AP) and lateral radiographs of displaced middle phalangeal neck fracture of the long finger in a 13-year-old male (a, b). Clinical examination demonstrating malrotation of the long finger (c), with elimination of the deformity after a closed reduction is performed (d). Intraoperative fluoroscopic AP (e) and lateral (f) images demonstrating reduction with two K-wires placed in oblique retrograde fashion.

- Subcondylar fossa reconstruction may be required if the above criteria are not met:
  - Incipient malunions, or partially healed malaligned fractures.
    - Treatment: Osteoclasis with percutaneous reduction and K-wire fixation.[8,12]

4. Nonunions

- Treatment:
  - Removal of sclerotic bone, reduction, and K-wire fixation with or without bone grafting may be required.[10]

III. Condyle Fractures

A. Background

- Intra-articular
- May present with various patterns, including:
  - Unicondylar/intracondylar fractures
  - Bicondylar/transcondylar fractures
  - Lateral avulsion fractures
  - Shearing fractures
    - Separate the articular surface and subchondral bone from the remaining phalanx.[2]
- Most fractures are displaced.
- Subluxation or dislocation of the associated interphalangeal joint is also common.[17]

B. Mechanism of Injury

- Direct axial force on the digit
- Avulsion from the collateral ligaments
- Shearing of the subchondral bone[2,3]
- In children, these forces may result from:
  - Jamming of finger from a ball
  - Fall
  - Crush
  - Torsional injury[18]

C. Evaluation Considerations

- Three radiographic views of the finger:
  - AP view
    - Fracture may not always be evident on this view.
  - Lateral view
    - Double density sign may sometimes be present, representing the displaced fractured condyle.[2,3]
  - Oblique view
    - Often most useful.

D. Treatment

- Anatomic reduction with operative intervention typically required.[19]

1. Closed/Percutaneous Reduction and K-Wire Fixation

- Indications
  - May suffice for acute injuries.[2,20]
- Technique
  - Obtain an oblique view in the operating room:
    - Oftentimes the fracture can appear reduced on AP and lateral imaging.
    - Only the oblique view may demonstrate continued displacement.
  - Closed reduction via a nonpenetrating towel clip or percutaneous reduction with a pin.
  - Immobilize hand with pins kept in place for 4 weeks:[21]
    - Sometimes healing is delayed because these fractures are intra-articular.
    - Patients may need further immobilization after pin removal.

2. Open Reduction and Fixation

- Indications
  - Bone is entrapped in the subcondylar fossa, blocking flexion.
  - Significant displacement (▶ Fig. 25.5).[2]
- Technique
  - Preserve soft tissue (i.e., the collateral ligaments).
    - Open management incurs a higher risk for avascular necrosis.[2,21]
  - Pins or mini screws can be used for fixation.
  - Immobilization via casting to protect the fixation.

E. Complications

- Delayed treatment:
  - Makes anatomic reduction more challenging and places the patient at higher risk for avascular necrosis.
  - Presentation is often delayed due to failed recognition by the patient's family and/ or the initial treating physician.[22,23]
  - Delays of up to 2 weeks can still generally achieve good outcomes.[22]
- Malunion and deformity:
  - Poor remodeling potential of condyle fractures due to the significant distance from the phalangeal physis.
  - Osteotomy of a condyle malunion should not be performed for several months due to high risk of avascular necrosis:
    - Delayed intervention reduces the risk of iatrogenically induced AVN.[2,23]
    - Families should be counseled on these risks.

IV. Seymour's Fractures

A. Background

- Distal phalanx fractures with a juxta-epiphyseal or Salter-Harris I or II pattern.[24]

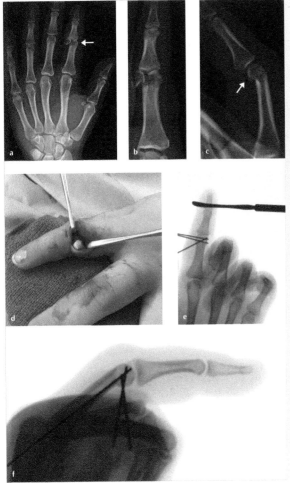

Fig. 25.5 Anteroposterior (AP) (a), oblique (b), and lateral (c) radiographs demonstrating a displaced proximal phalanx ulnar condyle fracture of the index finger in a 14-year-old female. Clinical image (d) demonstrating the widely displaced and rotated fragment. Intraoperative fluoroscopy AP (e) and lateral (f) images demonstrating good alignment of the fracture, maintained with K-wire fixation (e, f).

- The dorsally displaced fragment may lacerate the nail bed, creating an open fracture.[3,25]
- Imperative to recognize these injuries and employ the current principles of open fracture management.

B. Treatment

- In general, thorough irrigation and debridement, anatomic reduction and stabilization, and timely antibiotics required.[26]
- Bedside nail plate removal, exposure of the germinal matrix by incising the eponychium, irrigation and debridement (I&D), fracture reduction, with or without nail bed laceration repair, and immobilization (▶ Fig. 25.6).
  - ○ Indications:
    - – If closed reduction can be performed.
    - – Patient able to tolerate.

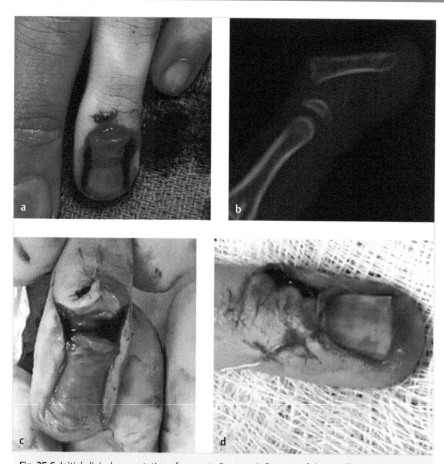

Fig. 25.6 Initial clinical presentation of an acute Seymour's fracture of the ring finger of a 10-year-old boy (a). Lateral radiograph demonstrating significant displacement (b). The eponychium must be incised and nail plate removed. The germinal matrix must be extracted from the growth plate, the wound thoroughly irrigated, and then the fracture reduced. This can be performed in the emergency department with a digital block with or without sedation (c). The nail plate can be replaced beneath the eponychial fold to help stabilize the reduction. The eponychium is closed with absorbable suture and a splint or cast is applied (d).

- ○ Techniques:
  - – May be performed at bedside in emergency department (ED).
  - – Local anesthesia via digital block.
  - – Conscious sedation if patient unable to tolerate digital block.
  - – Replace removed nail plate beneath the eponychial fold to protect the repair and fracture reduction when possible.
- • Formal I&D, open reduction, and K-wire fixation in operating room.
  - ○ Indications:
    - – If bedside reduction in ED is unsuccessful or remains unstable.[27,28,29]

– Some prefer to manage all open Seymour's fractures in the operating room under general anesthesia, as these patients are often very young.[30]
- Antibiotics
  ○ Patients may receive a dose of intravenous antibiotics in the ED.
  ○ All should be sent home with a course of oral antibiotics.

C. Complications

- Post-traumatic nail deformities
  ○ Reduce risk with meticulous primary repair with removal of the nail plate for exposure of the nail bed and germinal matrix:[31]
    – Removal of the nail plate may result in fracture instability in Seymour's fractures.[24,32,33]
    – However, removal is necessary for thorough I&D and primary repair of the nail bed laceration.[27]
- Osteomyelitis
  ○ Risk is increased with failure to recognize these injuries as open fractures.
  ○ Leads to increased likelihood of physeal arrest:
    – Premature physeal closure is often secondary to infection rather than direct injury to the growth plate.[32,33,34]
- Persistent mallet-type deformity.[35]

V. Mallet Injuries

A. Background

- Injuries of the extensor mechanism at the distal interphalangeal (DIP) joint.
- Can be isolated soft tissue injuries or avulsion-type bony fractures (▶ Fig. 25.7).
- Extensor mechanism is disrupted, so patients present with a flexed DIP joint:
  ○ Hence the "mallet" deformity and extensor lag.

B. Mechanism of Injury

- Direct force at the fingertip causing excessive flexion on an extended finger:
  ○ Often a jamming type injury from sports (i.e., when a ball directly impacts the fingertip[36]).

C. Treatment

- Goal is to restore active DIP joint extension and prevent secondary deformity.

1. Extension Splinting Alone

- Indications
  ○ Vast majority of children.
  ○ Regardless of extent of DIP joint articular surface involvement of the fracture (▶ Fig. 25.8).[36]
- Techniques
  ○ Around-the-clock wear of the orthosis for 6 to 8 weeks.

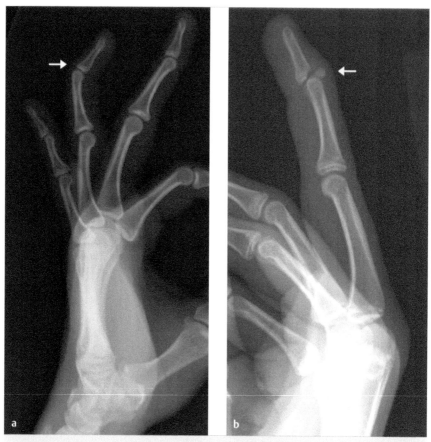

Fig. 25.7 Soft tissue mallet finger injury in ring finger of a 16-year-old male **(a)**. Bony mallet injury in the long finger of 15-year-old male **(b)**.

- Nonadherence to immobilization is associated with residual DIP joint extensor lag and complications.[36]

2. Operative Pin Fixation

- Indications
  - ○ Controversial
    - Insufficient evidence to determine when surgical intervention is required.[37]
  - ○ For adults, some report percentage of involvement of the DIP joint articular surface[38,39] and presence of distal phalanx subluxation or displacement as indications for operative fixation.[40,41,42]
    - Others recommend conservative management for almost all cases with extension splinting alone.[43,44,45,46,47]

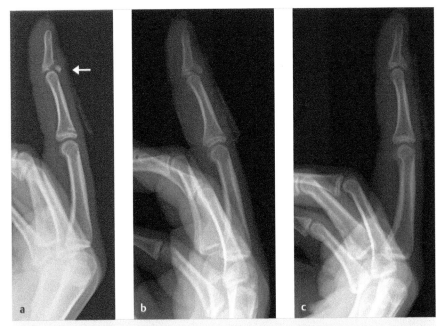

Fig. 25.8 Bony mallet finger injury in a 15-year-old male, splinted in extension on presentation **(a)**; 3.5 weeks after initiation of extension splinting **(b)**; 7 weeks after initiation of splinting shows a healed fracture with remodeling at the joint surface **(c)**. Clinically, he had no pain or extensor lag.

VI. Bony Thumb Ulnar Collateral Ligament (UCL) Injuries

A. Background

- Referred to as pediatric skier's thumb.
- Involves a Salter-Harris III intra-articular avulsion fracture at the UCL insertion at the proximal phalanx epiphysis of the thumb (▶ Fig. 25.9).
  - Thumb UCL injuries in children usually have bony involvement.[2]
- Presents with pain at the ulnar aspect of the joint as well as valgus instability of the thumb.

B. Mechanism of Injury

- Hyperabduction of the thumb.
- Avulsion typically occurs rather than an isolated ligamentous rupture.
- This destabilizes the metacarpophalangeal (MCP) joint.

C. Pathoanatomy

- Avulsion fracture eliminates the structural contribution of both components of the UCL:

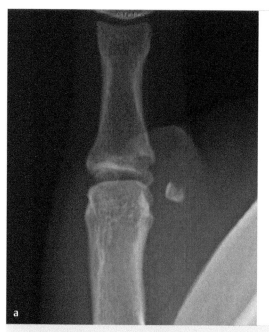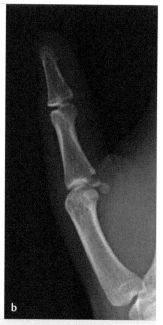

Fig. 25.9 (a, b) Bony ulnar collateral ligament (UCL) injury (avulsion fracture) of the thumb proximal phalanx in a 16-year-old male.

- ○ Proper collateral ligaments:
  - – Normally resist valgus load in flexion.
- ○ Accessory collateral ligaments:
  - – Normally resist valgus loads in extension.
- In bony injuries, the actual UCL is usually intact in children:
  - ○ Ligament is attached to the avulsed bony fragment.
  - ○ Cases of isolated UCL rupture in children have been reported in the literature:[48,49]
    - – These cases can be operatively managed by suturing the ligament to its bony insertion through various techniques.

D. Treatment

1. Immobilization Alone

- Indications
  - ○ Nondisplaced UCL avulsion fracture.
- Techniques
  - ○ Short arm thumb spica cast 4 to 6 weeks.[50]

2. Closed Reduction and Percutaneous Pinning (CRPP) or Open Reduction and Internal Fixation (ORIF)

- Indications
  - ○ Displaced fractures.[2,21]

- Techniques:
  - Incision over the ulnar aspect of the thumb MCP joint to visualize the reduction (▶ Fig. 25.10).
  - Reduce fracture and confirm intact UCL.
  - K-wires are employed to stabilize the fracture fragment, inserting from ulnar to radial.
  - Suture anchors, tension-band wiring, or screws may also be used for fixation:
    - Avoid injuring an open growth plate.[2,21,51]
  - Immobilize in cast for 4 weeks:
    - Pull pins at 4 weeks.
    - Can transition to a removable brace at this point.

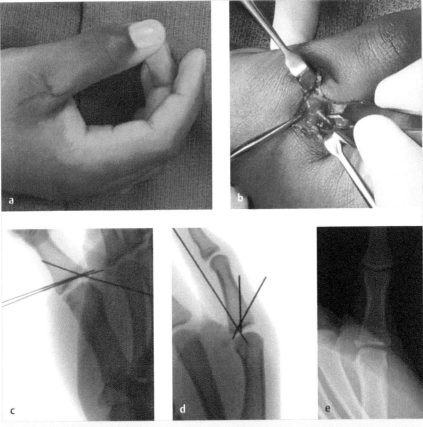

Fig. 25.10 S-shaped incision starting dorsally proximally and angling volarly distally at the thumb metacarpophalangeal joint (**a**). Facture fragment with 180 degrees of malrotation (cartilage surface facing distally) (**b**). Intraoperative fluoroscopy anteroposterior (AP) (**c**) and lateral (**d**) imaging demonstrating K-wires stabilizing the fracture fragment. AP image demonstrates almost complete radiographic healing at 5 weeks, although the patient was clinically healed without any pain with deep pressure (**e**).

3. Formal Therapy

• Not required for most patients to regain full function and return to prior activity levels.

VII. Conclusion

• Pediatric hand fractures are common injuries with unique challenges in both their recognition and treatment. Although the substantial skeletal healing potential of children generally affords good clinical outcomes, they also require appropriate timely management in order to prevent complications and deformity. Therefore, it is imperative for providers to accurately identify these fractures and recognize when a hand surgeon should be involved. Operative interventions pose distinct challenges, with various fracture patterns demanding unique indications and displaying varying pitfalls. Counseling of patients' families is also crucial, as success of treatment may be dependent on adherence to rehabilitation and immobilization protocols.

References

[1] Al-Qattan MM, Al-Zahrani K, Al-Boukai AA. The relative incidence of fractures at the base of the proximal phalanx of the fingers in children. J Hand Surg Eur Vol. 2008; 33(4):465–468

[2] Cornwall R, Ricchetti ET. Pediatric phalanx fractures: unique challenges and pitfalls. Clin Orthop Relat Res. 2006; 445(445):146–156

[3] Nellans KW, Chung KC. Pediatric hand fractures. Hand Clin. 2013; 29(4):569–578

[4] Beatty E, Light TR, Belsole RJ, Ogden JA. Wrist and hand skeletal injuries in children. Hand Clin. 1990; 6 (4):723–738

[5] Al-Qattan MM, Al-Munif DS, AlHammad AK, AlFayez DI, Hanouneh S. The outcome of management of "troublesome" vs "non-troublesome" phalangeal neck fractures in children less than 2 years of age. J Plast Surg Hand Surg. 2016; 50(2):93–101

[6] Al-Qattan MM. Nonunion and avascular necrosis following phalangeal neck fractures in children. J Hand Surg Am. 2010; 35(8):1269–1274

[7] Barton NJ. Fractures of the phalanges of the hand in children. Hand. 1979; 11(2):134–143

[8] Matzon JL, Cornwall R. A stepwise algorithm for surgical treatment of type II displaced pediatric phalangeal neck fractures. J Hand Surg Am. 2014; 39(3):467–473

[9] Al-Qattan MM. Phalangeal neck fractures in children: classification and outcome in 66 cases. J Hand Surg [Br]. 2001; 26(2):112–121

[10] Al-Qattan MM, Al-Qattan AM. A review of phalangeal neck fractures in children. Injury. 2015; 46 (6):935–944

[11] Leonard MH, Dubravcik P. Management of fractured fingers in the child. Clin Orthop Relat Res. 1970; 73 (73):160–168

[12] Waters PM, Taylor BA, Kuo AY. Percutaneous reduction of incipient malunion of phalangeal neck fractures in children. J Hand Surg Am. 2004; 29(4):707–711

[13] Londner J, Salazard B, Gay A, Samson P, Legré R. [A new technique of intrafocal pinning for phalangeal neck fractures in children]. Chir Main. 2008; 27(1):20–25

[14] Topouchian V, Fitoussi F, Jehanno P, Frajman JM, Mazda K, Penneçot GF. Treatment of phalangeal neck fractures in children: technical suggestion. Chir Main. 2003; 22(6):299–304

[15] Kang HJ, Sung SY, Ha JW, Yoon HK, Hahn SB. Operative treatment for proximal phalangeal neck fractures of the finger in children. Yonsei Med J. 2005; 46(4):491–495

[16] Cornwall R, Waters PM. Remodeling of phalangeal neck fracture malunions in children: case report. J Hand Surg Am. 2004; 29(3):458–461

[17] Graham T, Waters P. Fractures and dislocations of the hand and carpus in children. In: Beaty J, Kasser J, eds. Rockwood and Wilkins' Fractures in Children. 5 ed. Philadelphia, PA: Lippincott, William & Wilkins; 2001:269–379

[18] Freeland AE, Sud V. Unicondylar and bicondylar proximal phalangeal fractures. J Am Soc Surg Hand. 2001; 1 (1):14–24

[19] Weiss AP, Hastings H, II. Distal unicondylar fractures of the proximal phalanx. J Hand Surg Am. 1993; 18 (4):594–599

[20] Markeson D, Iyer S. A simple technique for the reduction of phalangeal condylar fractures in children. Ann R Coll Surg Engl. 2012; 94(2):138

[21] Abzug JM, Dua K, Bauer AS, Cornwall R, Wyrick TO. Pediatric phalanx fractures. J Am Acad Orthop Surg. 2016; 24(11):e174–e183

[22] Shewring DJ, Miller AC, Ghandour A. Condylar fractures of the proximal and middle phalanges. J Hand Surg Eur Vol. 2015; 40(1):51–58

[23] Puckett BN, Gaston RG, Peljovich AE, Lourie GM, Floyd WE, III. Remodeling potential of phalangeal distal condylar malunions in children. J Hand Surg Am. 2012; 37(1):34–41

[24] Seymour N. Juxta-epiphysial fracture of the terminal phalanx of the finger. J Bone Joint Surg Br. 1966; 48 (2):347–349

[25] Lindor RA, Sadosty AT. Images in emergency medicine. A jammed finger and bloody nail. Seymour fracture. Ann Emerg Med. 2014; 63(6):656–677

[26] Pape HC, Webb LX. History of open wound and fracture treatment. J Orthop Trauma. 2008; 22(10) Suppl: S133–S134

[27] Reyes BA, Ho CA. The high risk of infection with delayed treatment of open Seymour fractures: Salter-Harris I/II or juxta-epiphyseal fractures of the distal phalanx with associated nailbed laceration. J Pediatr Orthop. 2017; 37(4):247–253

[28] Al-Qattan MM. Extra-articular transverse fractures of the base of the distal phalanx (Seymour's fracture) in children and adults. J Hand Surg [Br]. 2001; 26(3):201–206

[29] Krusche-Mandl I, Köttstorfer J, Thalhammer G, Aldrian S, Erhart J, Platzer P. Seymour fractures: retrospective analysis and therapeutic considerations. J Hand Surg Am. 2013; 38(2):258–264

[30] Abzug JM, Kozin SH. Seymour fractures. J Hand Surg Am. 2013; 38(11):2267–2270, quiz 2270

[31] Inglefield CJ, D'Arcangelo M, Kolhe PS. Injuries to the nail bed in childhood. J Hand Surg [Br]. 1995; 20 (2):258–261

[32] Ganayem M, Edelson G. Base of distal phalanx fracture in children: a mallet finger mimic. J Pediatr Orthop. 2005; 25(4):487–489

[33] Wood VE. Fractures of the hand in children. Orthop Clin North Am. 1976; 7(3):527–542

[34] Engber WD, Clancy WG. Traumatic avulsion of the finger nail associated with injury to the phalangeal epiphyseal plate. J Bone Joint Surg Am. 1978; 60(5):713–714

[35] Lankachandra M, Wells CR, Cheng CJ, Hutchison RL. Complications of distal phalanx fractures in children. J Hand Surg Am. 2017; 42(7):574.e1–574.e6

[36] Lin JS, Samora JB. Outcomes of splinting in pediatric mallet finger. J Hand Surg Am. 2018; 43(11):1041.e1–1041.e9

[37] Lin JS, Samora JB. Surgical and nonsurgical management of mallet finger: a systematic review. J Hand Surg Am. 2018; 43(2):146–163.e2

[38] Hamas RS, Horrell ED, Pierret GP. Treatment of mallet finger due to intra-articular fracture of the distal phalanx. J Hand Surg Am. 1978; 3(4):361–363

[39] Houpt P, Dijkstra R, Storm van Leeuwen JB. Fowler's tenotomy for mallet deformity. J Hand Surg [Br]. 1993; 18(4):499–500

[40] McCue FC, Abbott JL. The treatment of mallet finger and boutonniere deformities. Va Med Mon (1918). 1967; 94(10):623–628

[41] Stark HH, Gainor BJ, Ashworth CR, Zemel NP, Rickard TA. Operative treatment of intra-articular fractures of the dorsal aspect of the distal phalanx of digits. J Bone Joint Surg Am. 1987; 69(6):892–896

[42] Takami H, Takahashi S, Ando M. Operative treatment of mallet finger due to intra-articular fracture of the distal phalanx. Arch Orthop Trauma Surg. 2000; 120(1–2):9–13

[43] Wehbé MA, Schneider LH. Mallet fractures. J Bone Joint Surg Am. 1984; 66(5):658–669

[44] Weber P, Segmüller H. Non-surgical treatment of mallet finger fractures involving more than one third of the joint surface: 10 cases. Handchir Mikrochir Plast Chir. 2008; 40(3):145–148

[45] Kalainov DM, Hoepfner PE, Hartigan BJ, Carroll C, IV, Genuario J. Nonsurgical treatment of closed mallet finger fractures. J Hand Surg Am. 2005; 30(3):580–586

[46] Facca S, Nonnenmacher J, Liverneaux P. Treatment of mallet finger with dorsal nail glued splint: retrospective analysis of 270 cases. Rev Chir Orthop Reparatrice Appar Mot. 2007; 93(7):682–689

[47] Salazar Botero S, Hidalgo Diaz JJ, Benaïda A, Collon S, Facca S, Liverneaux PA. Review of acute traumatic closed mallet finger injuries in adults. Arch Plast Surg. 2016; 43(2):134–144

[48] Davies MB, Wright JE, Edwards MS. True skier's thumb in childhood. Injury. 2002; 33(2):186–187

[49] White GM. Ligamentous avulsion of the ulnar collateral ligament of the thumb of a child. J Hand Surg Am. 1986; 11(5):669–672

[50] Kocher MS, Waters PM, Micheli LJ. Upper extremity injuries in the paediatric athlete. Sports Med. 2000; 30 (2):117–135

[51] Green DP, Wolfe SW. Green's operative hand surgery. Saunders/Elsevier; 2011

Index

Note: Page numbers set **bold** or *italic* indicate headings or figures, respectively.

Index